SO-ADY-385

1998 Guidelines for Treatment of Sexually Transmitted Diseases

Morbidity and Mortality Weekly Report
January 23, 1998
Vol. 47, No. RR-1

U.S. Department of Health and Human Services
Centers for Disease Control and Prevention

International Medical Publishing, Inc.

Compliments of

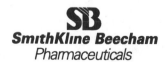

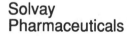

Neither the CDC nor the U.S. Department of Health and Human Services endorses any particular organization or its activities, products, or services.

Other titles from International Medical Publishing
    The Intern Pocket Survival Guide
    The Surgical Intern Pocket Survival Guide
    The CCU Intern Pocket Survival Guide
    The ER Intern Pocket Survival Guide
    The ICU Intern Pocket Survival Guide
    The Oncology Intern Pocket Survival Guide

    The EKG Pocket Survival Guide
    The ACLS Pocket Survival Guide
    The PALS Pocket Survival Guide

    The Pocket Guide to Eponyms and Subtle Signs of Disease
    How to be a Truly Excellent Junior Medical Student

    Clinician's Handbook of Preventive Services, 2nd edition
    Guide to Clinical Preventive Services, 2nd edition
    Health Information for International Travel 1996-97
    JNC VI Report on Hypertension
    First Aid

1998 Guidelines for Treatment of Sexually Transmitted Diseases is provided in its entirety. International Medical Publishing, Inc. provides no warranty for the data or the opinions expressed herein.

The material contained within is in the public domain.

First Printing.

1998 Guidelines for Treatment of Sexually Transmitted Diseases
U.S. Department of Health and Human Services
Centers for Disease Control and Prevention (CDC)
International Medical Publishing, Inc.
ISBN 1-883205-45-X

Other titles are available mail order from:
    International Medical Publishing, Inc., 13017 Wisteria Drive, #313, Germantown, MD 20874

Order on the web from:
    http://www.intlmedpub.com

Published by International Medical Publishing, Inc., P.O. Box 479, McLean, VA 22101-0479
    tel 703-519-0807
    fax 703-519-0806
    http://www.intlmedpub.com

Printed in the United States of America

The *MMWR* series of publications is published by the Epidemiology Program Office, Centers for Disease Control and Prevention (CDC), U.S. Department of Health and Human Services, Atlanta, GA 30333.

SUGGESTED CITATION

Centers for Disease Control and Prevention. 1998 Guidelines for treatment of sexually transmitted diseases. MMWR 1998;47(No. RR-1):[inclusive page numbers].

Centers for Disease Control and Prevention .... David Satcher, M.D., Ph.D.
Director

Dixie E. Snider, M.D., M.P.H.
Associate Director for Science

The material in this report was prepared for publication by:

National Center for HIV, STD and TB Prevention .... Helene D. Gayle, M.D., M.P.H.
Director

Division of Sexually Transmitted
Diseases Prevention ....Judith Wasserheit, M.D., M.P.H.
Director

The production of this report as an *MMWR* serial publication was coordinated in:

Epidemiology Program Office.................................... Stephen B. Thacker, M.D., M.Sc.
Director

Richard A. Goodman, M.D., M.P.H.
Editor, MMWR *Series*

Office of Scientific and Health Communications (proposed)

Recommendations and Reports................................... Suzanne M. Hewitt, M.P.A.
Managing Editor

Lanette B. Wolcott
Project Editor

Morie M. Higgins
Peter M. Jenkins
Visual Information Specialist

Use of trade names and commercial sources is for identification only and does not imply endorsement by the U.S. Department of Health and Human Services.

Contents

Abbreviations Used in This Publication

ACIP	Advisory Committee on Immunization Practices
ACOG	American College of Obstetricians and Gynecologists
ACS	American Cancer Society
AIDS	Acquired immunodeficiency syndrome
anti-HBc	Antibody to hepatitis B core antigen
ASCUS	Atypical squamous cells of undetermined significance
BCA	Bichloroacetic acid
BV	Bacterial vaginosis
CBC	Complete blood count
CI	Confidence interval
CIN	Cervical intraepithelial neoplasia
CMV	Cytomegalovirus
CSF	Cerebrospinal fluid
d4t	Stavudine
ddC	Dideoxycytodine
ddl	Didanosine
DGI	Disseminated gonococcal infection
DNA	Deoxyribonucleic acid
EIA	Enzyme immunoassay
FDA	Food and Drug Administration
FTA-ABS	Fluorescent treponemal antibody absorbed
GISP	Gonococcal Isolate Surveillance Project
HAV	Hepatitis A virus
HBIG	Hepatitis B immune globulin
HBsAg	Hepatitis B surface antigen
HbeAg	Hepatitis B e Antigen
HBV	Hepatitis B virus
HIV	Human immunodeficiency virus
HPV	Human papillomavirus
HSV	Herpes simplex virus
IFA	Immunofluorescence assay
IG	Immune globulin
IM	Intramuscularly
IV	Intravenous or intravenously
KOH	Potassium hydroxide
LGV	Lymphogranuloma venereum
MAC	*Mycobacterium avium* complex
MIC	Minimum inhibitory concentration
MPC	Mucopurulent cervicitis
MHA-TP	Microhemagglutination assay for antibody to *Treponema pallidum*
NGU	Nongonococcal urethritis

Abbreviations Used in This Publication — Continued

OTC	Over-the-counter
Pap	Papanicolaou
PCP	*Pneumocystis carinii* pneumonia
PCR	Polymerase chain reaction
PID	Pelvic inflammatory disease
PPD	Purified protein derivative
PPV	Positive predictive value
QRNG	Quinolone-resistant *Neisseria gonorrhoeae*
RNA	Ribonucleic acid
RPR	Rapid plasma reagin
RVVC	Recurrent vulvovaginal candidiasis
SAQ	Saquinavir
SIL	Squamous intraepithelial lesions
STD	Sexually transmitted disease
TB	Tuberculosis
TCA	Trichloroacetic acid
TE	Toxoplasmic encephalitis
TST	Tuberculin skin test
VDRL	Venereal Disease Research Laboratory
VVC	Vulvovaginal candidiasis
WB	Western blot
WBC	White blood cell
ZDV	Zidovudine
3TC	Lamivudine

Expert Consultants

Chairman: David Atkins, M.D., M.P.H., Agency for Health Care Policy and Research; **Presenters:** Michael H. Augenbraun, M.D., State University of New York Health Science Center at Brooklyn, NY; Karl Beutner, M.D., Ph.D., Solano Dermatology, Vallejo, CA; Gail A. Bolan, M.D., San Francisco Department of Public Health and University of California at San Francisco; Willard Cates, Jr., M.D., M.P.H., Family Health International, Research Triangle Park, NC; Anne M. Rompalo, M.D., Johns Hopkins University, Baltimore; Pablo J. Sanchez, M.D., Southwestern Medical Center at Dallas; Bradley Stoner, M.D., Ph.D., Washington University School of Medicine, St. Louis, MO; Anna Wald, M.D., M.P.H., University of Washington, Seattle; Cheryl K. Walker, M.D., University of California at Irvine; George D. Wendel, M.D., Southwestern Medical Center at Dallas; Jonathan M. Zenilman, M.D., Johns Hopkins University, Baltimore. **Moderators:** King K. Holmes, M.D., Ph.D., Center for AIDS and STDs, University of Washington, Seattle; Edward W. Hook, III, M.D., University of Alabama at Birmingham School of Medicine; A. Eugene Washington, M.D., M.Sc., University of California at San Francisco. **Rapporteurs:** John M. Douglas, Jr., M.D., Denver Department of Public Health and University of Colorado Health Science Center; Margaret R. Hammerschlag, M.D., State University of New York Health Science Center; David H. Martin, M.D., Louisiana State University Medical Center, New Orleans. **Consultants:** Adaora A. Adimora, M.D., M.P.H., University of North Carolina at Chapel Hill; Virginia A. Caine, M.D., Marion County Health Department, Indianapolis; Laura T. Gutman, M.D., Duke University, Durham, NC; H. Hunter Handsfield, M.D., Seattle-King County Department of Public Health and University of Washington, Seattle; Robert B. Jones, M.D., Ph.D., Indiana University, Indianapolis; Franklyn N. Judson, M.D., Denver Department of Health; William M. McCormack, M.D., State University of New York Health Science Center at Brooklyn; Daniel M. Musher, M.D., Baylor College of Medicine, Houston; Newton G. Osborne, M.D., M.P.H., Howard University Hospital, Washington, DC; Robert T. Rolfs, Jr., M.D., Utah Department of Health; Lawrence L. Sanders, Jr., M.D., Southwest Hospital and Medical Center, Atlanta; Jane R. Schwebke, M.D., University of Alabama at Birmingham School of Medicine; Jack D. Sobel, M.D., Wayne State University School of Medicine, Detroit; David E. Soper, M.D., Medical University of South Carolina, Charleston; Walter E. Stamm, M.D., University of Washington; Lawrence R. Stanberry, M.D., Ph.D., Children's Hospital, Cincinnati; Felicia H. Stewart, M.D., Kaiser Family Foundation, Menlo Park, CA; Richard L. Sweet, M.D., Magee-Women's Hospital, Pittsburgh.

Other Expert Consultants (did not attend meeting): Susan Blank, M.D., New York City Department of Health; Sharon L. Hillier, Ph.D., University of Pittsburgh; Penelope J. Hitchcock, D.V.M., M.S., National Institutes of Health; Paul N. Zenker, M.D., M.P.H., Franklin Primary Health, Mobile, AL.

Liaison Participants: Dennis J. Barbour, J.D., Association of Reproductive Health Professionals; Joan R. Cates, American Social Health Association; JoAnne Doherty, Health Canada, Ontario; Robert G. Harmon, M.D., M.P.H., United Health Care; Kate L. Heilpern, M.D., American College of Emergency Physicians; John J. Henning, Ph.D., American Medical Association; K. King Holmes, M.D., Ph.D., Infectious

Diseases Society of America; John N. Krieger, M.D., American Urological Association; Marshall Kubota, M.D., American Academy of Family Practice; Noni E. MacDonald, M.D., American Academy of Pediatrics; Gary A. Richwald, M.D., M.P.H., National Coalition of STD Directors; Helen J. Sawyer, R.N., Georgia Department of Human Resources; Stanley X. Shapiro, M.D., Regional Laboratory and Infectious Disease Committee, Kaiser Permanente, Panorama City, CA; Donald Sutherland, M.D., Health Canada; Steve K. Tyring, M.D., Ph.D., American Academy of Dermatology; C. Johannes van Dam, M.D., World Health Organization; Fernando Zacarias, M.D., M.P.H., Pan American Health Organization, World Health Organization.

CDC/Division of STD Prevention (DSTDP)/STD Treatment Guidelines 1997 Project Coordinators: Kimberly A. Workowski, M.D.; John S. Moran, M.D.; **Co-Chair:** Michael E. St. Louis, M.D.; **Co-Moderator:** Katherine M. Stone, M.D.; **Presenters:** Consuelo M. Beck-Sague, M.D., National Center for Infectious Diseases (NCID); M. Riduan Joesoef, M.D., Ph.D., M.P.H.; Mary L. Kamb, M.D., M.P.H., Division of HIV/AIDS Prevention (DHAP); Jonathan E. Kaplan, M.D., NCID; H. Trent MacKay, M.D., M.P.H.; Michael M. McNeil, M.D., M.P.H., NCID; Allyn K. Nakashima, M.D., DHAP; George P. Schmid, M.D., M.Sc.; **Consultants:** Sevgi O. Aral, Ph.D.; Stuart M. Berman, M.D.; Donald F. Dowda; Brian R. Edlin, M.D., DHAP; Helene D. Gayle, M.D., M.P.H., National Center for HIV, STD, and TB Prevention (NCHSTP); Robert S. Janssen, M.D., DHAP; Wanda K. Jones, Dr.P.H., Office of Women's Health; William J. Kassler, M.D., M.P.H.; Nancy C. Lee, M.D., DHAP; Beth Macke, Ph.D.; Frank J. Mahoney, M.D., NCID; Phillip I. Nieberg, M.D., M.P.H., NCHSTP; Herbert B. Peterson, M.D., National Center for Chronic Disease Prevention and Health Promotion (NCCDPHP); Martha F. Rogers, M.D., DHAP; William E. Secor, Ph.D., NCID; Dawn K. Smith, M.D., DHAP; Ronald O. Valdiserri, M.D., M.P.H., NCHSTP; Judith N. Wasserheit, M.D., M.P.H.; Lynne S. Wilcox, M.D., NCCDPHP; **Support Staff:** Cynthia Ford, Contractor; Deborah McElroy; Garrett K. Mallory.

1998 Guidelines for Treatment of
Sexually Transmitted Diseases

Summary

These guidelines for the treatment of patients who have sexually transmitted diseases (STDs) were developed by CDC staff members after consultation with a group of invited experts who met in Atlanta on February 10–12, 1997. The information in this report updates the "1993 Sexually Transmitted Diseases Treatment Guidelines" (MMWR 1993;42[no. RR-14]). Included are new recommendations for treatment of primary and recurrent genital herpes and management of pelvic inflammatory disease; a new patient-applied medication for treatment of genital warts; and a revised approach to the management of victims of sexual assault. Revised sections describe the evaluation of urethritis and the diagnostic evaluation of congenital syphilis. These guidelines also include expanded sections concerning STDs among infants, children, and pregnant women and the management of patients who have asymptomatic human immunodeficiency virus infection, genital warts, and genital herpes. Guidelines are provided for vaccine-preventable STDs, including recommendations for the use of hepatitis A and hepatitis B vaccines.

INTRODUCTION

Physicians and other health-care providers have a critical role in preventing and treating sexually transmitted diseases (STDs). These recommendations for the treatment of STDs, which were developed by CDC staff members in consultation with a group of invited experts, are intended to assist with that effort.

This report was produced through a multi-stage process. Beginning in the spring of 1996, CDC personnel and invited experts systematically reviewed literature concerning each of the major STDs, focusing on information that had become available since the "1993 Sexually Transmitted Diseases Treatment Guidelines" (*MMWR* 1993;42[no. RR-14]) were published. Background papers were written and tables of evidence constructed summarizing the type of study (e.g., randomized controlled trial or case series), study population and setting, treatments or other interventions, outcome measures assessed, reported findings, and weaknesses and biases in study design and analysis. For these reviews, published abstracts and peer-reviewed journal articles were considered. A draft document was developed on the basis of the reviews.

In February 1997, invited consultants assembled in Atlanta for a 3-day meeting. CDC personnel and invited experts presented the key questions on STD treatment suggested from the literature reviews and presented the information available to answer those questions. Where relevant, the questions focused on four principal outcomes of STD therapy: a) microbiologic cure, b) alleviation of signs and symptoms, c) prevention of sequelae, and d) prevention of transmission. Cost-effectiveness and other advantages (e.g., single-dose formulations and directly observed therapy) of specific regimens also were considered. The consultants then assessed whether the questions identified were appropriate, ranked them in order of priority, and attempted to arrive at answers using the available evidence. In addition, the consultants evaluated the quality of evidence supporting the answers on the basis of the number, type, and quality of the studies.

In several areas, the process diverged from that described previously. The sections concerning adolescents, congenital syphilis, and partner notification were reviewed by other CDC experts on prevention of STDs and human immunodeficiency virus (HIV) infection. The recommendations for STD screening during pregnancy were developed after CDC staff reviewed the published recommendations of other expert groups. The sections concerning early HIV infection are a compilation of recommendations developed by CDC experts in HIV infection. The sections on hepatitis B virus (HBV) (*1*) and hepatitis A virus (HAV) (*2*) infections are based on previously published recommendations of the Advisory Committee on Immunization Practices (ACIP).

Throughout this report, the evidence used as the basis for specific recommendations is discussed briefly. More comprehensive, annotated discussions of such evidence will appear in background papers that will be published in 1998. When more than one therapeutic regimen is recommended, the sequence is alphabetized unless there is priority of choice (i.e., based on efficacy, convenience, and cost). Almost all recommended regimens have similar efficacy and similar rates of intolerance or toxicity unless otherwise specified.

These recommendations were developed in consultation with experts whose experience is primarily with the treatment of patients in public STD clinics. Nevertheless, these recommendations also should be applicable to other patient-care settings, including family planning clinics, private physicians' offices, managed care organizations, and other primary-care facilities. When using these guidelines, the disease prevalence and other characteristics of the medical practice setting should be considered. These recommendations should be regarded as a source of clinical guidance and not as standards or inflexible rules.

These recommendations focus on the treatment and counseling of individual patients and do not address other community services and interventions that are important in STD/HIV prevention. Clinical and laboratory diagnoses are described when such information is related to therapy. For a more comprehensive discussion of diagnosis, refer to CDC's *Sexually Transmitted Diseases Clinical Practice Guidelines, 1991* (*3*).

CLINICAL PREVENTION GUIDELINES

The prevention and control of STDs is based on five major concepts: first, education of those at risk on ways to reduce the risk for STDs; second, detection of asymptomatically infected persons and of symptomatic persons unlikely to seek diagnostic and treatment services; third, effective diagnosis and treatment of infected persons; fourth, evaluation, treatment, and counseling of sex partners of persons who are infected with an STD; and fifth, preexposure vaccination of persons at risk for vaccine-preventable STDs. Although this report focuses primarily on the clinical aspects of STD control, prevention of STDs is based on changing the sexual behaviors that place persons at risk for infection. Moreover, because STD control activities reduce the likelihood of transmission to sex partners, prevention for individuals constitutes prevention for the community.

Clinicians have the opportunity to provide client education and counseling and to participate in identifying and treating infected sex partners in addition to interrupting transmission by treating persons who have the curable bacterial and parasitic STDs. The ability of the health-care provider to obtain an accurate sexual history is crucial in prevention and control efforts. Guidance in obtaining a sexual history is available in the chapter "Sexuality and Reproductive Health" in *Contraceptive Technology, 16th edition* (*4*). The accurate diagnosis and timely reporting of STDs by the clinician is the basis for effective public health surveillance.

Prevention Messages

Preventing the spread of STDs requires that persons at risk for transmitting or acquiring infections change their behaviors. The essential first step is for the health-care provider to proactively include questions regarding the patient's sexual history as part of the clinical interview. When risk factors have been identified, the provider has an opportunity to deliver prevention messages. Counseling skills (i.e., respect, compassion, and a nonjudgmental attitude) are essential to the effective delivery of prevention messages. Techniques that can be effective in facilitating a rapport with the patient include using open-ended questions, using understandable language, and reassuring the patient that treatment will be provided regardless of considerations such as ability to pay, citizenship or immigration status, language spoken, or lifestyle.

Prevention messages should be tailored to the patient, with consideration given to the patient's specific risk factors for STDs. Messages should include a description of specific actions that the patient can take to avoid acquiring or transmitting STDs (e.g., abstinence from sexual activity if STD-related symptoms develop).

Sexual Transmission

The most effective way to prevent sexual transmission of HIV infection and other STDs is to avoid sexual intercourse with an infected partner. Counseling that provides information concerning abstinence from penetrative sexual intercourse is crucial for a) persons who are being treated for an STD or whose partners are undergoing treatment and b) persons who wish to avoid the possible consequences of sexual intercourse (e.g., STD/HIV and pregnancy). A more comprehensive discussion of abstinence is available in *Contraceptive Technology, 16th edition* (*4*).

- Both partners should get tested for STDs, including HIV, before initiating sexual intercourse.

- If a person chooses to have sexual intercourse with a partner whose infection status is unknown or who is infected with HIV or another STD, a new condom should be used for each act of intercourse.

Injecting-Drug Users

The following prevention messages are appropriate for injecting-drug users:

- Enroll or continue in a drug-treatment program.

- Do not, under any circumstances, use injection equipment (e.g., needles and syringes) that has been used by another person.

- If needles can be obtained legally in the community, obtain clean needles.

- Persons who continue to use injection equipment that has been used by other persons should first clean the equipment with bleach and water. (Disinfecting with bleach does not sterilize the equipment and does not guarantee that HIV is inactivated. However, for injecting-drug users, thoroughly and consistently cleaning injection equipment with bleach should reduce the rate of HIV transmission when equipment is shared.)

Preexposure Vaccination

Preexposure vaccination is one of the most effective methods used to prevent transmission of certain STDs. HBV infection frequently is sexually transmitted, and hepatitis B vaccination is recommended for all unvaccinated patients being evaluated for an STD. In the United States, hepatitis A vaccines from two manufacturers were licensed recently. Hepatitis A vaccination is recommended for several groups of patients who might seek treatment in STD clinics; such patients include homosexual or bisexual men and persons who use illegal drugs. Vaccine trials for other STDs are being conducted, and vaccines for these STDs may become available within the next several years.

Prevention Methods

Male Condoms

When used consistently and correctly, condoms are effective in preventing many STDs, including HIV infection. Multiple cohort studies, including those of serodiscordant sex partners, have demonstrated a strong protective effect of condom use against HIV infection. Because condoms do not cover all exposed areas, they may be more effective in preventing infections transmitted between mucosal surfaces than those transmitted by skin-to-skin contact. Condoms are regulated as medical devices and are subject to random sampling and testing by the Food and Drug Administration (FDA). Each latex condom manufactured in the United States is tested electronically for holes before packaging. Rates of condom breakage during sexual intercourse and withdrawal are low in the United States (i.e., usually two broken condoms per 100 condoms used). Condom failure usually results from inconsistent or incorrect use rather than condom breakage.

Patients should be advised that condoms must be used consistently and correctly to be highly effective in preventing STDs. Patients also should be instructed in the correct use of condoms. The following recommendations ensure the proper use of male condoms:

- Use a new condom with each act of sexual intercourse.
- Carefully handle the condom to avoid damaging it with fingernails, teeth, or other sharp objects.
- Put the condom on after the penis is erect and before genital contact with the partner.
- Ensure that no air is trapped in the tip of the condom.
- Ensure that adequate lubrication exists during intercourse, possibly requiring the use of exogenous lubricants.
- Use only water-based lubricants (e.g., K-Y Jelly™, Astroglide™, AquaLube™, and glycerin) with latex condoms. Oil-based lubricants (e.g., petroleum jelly, shortening, mineral oil, massage oils, body lotions, and cooking oil) can weaken latex.
- Hold the condom firmly against the base of the penis during withdrawal, and withdraw while the penis is still erect to prevent slippage.

Female Condoms

Laboratory studies indicate that the female condom (Reality™)—a lubricated polyurethane sheath with a ring on each end that is inserted into the vagina—is an effective mechanical barrier to viruses, including HIV. Other than one investigation of recurrent trichomoniasis, no clinical studies have been completed to evaluate the efficacy of female condoms in providing protection from STDs, including HIV. If used consistently and correctly, the female condom should substantially reduce the risk for STDs. When a male condom cannot be used appropriately, sex partners should consider using a female condom.

Condoms and Spermicides

Whether condoms lubricated with spermicides are more effective than other lubricated condoms in protecting against the transmission of HIV and other STDs has not been determined. Furthermore, spermicide-coated condoms have been associated with *Escherichia coli* urinary tract infection in young women. Whether condoms used with vaginal application of spermicide are more effective than condoms used without vaginal spermicides also has not been determined. Therefore, the consistent use of condoms, with or without spermicidal lubricant or vaginal application of spermicide, is recommended.

Vaginal Spermicides, Sponges, and Diaphragms

As demonstrated in several randomized controlled trials, vaginal spermicides used alone without condoms reduce the risk for cervical gonorrhea and chlamydia. However, vaginal spermicides offer no protection against HIV infection, and spermicides are not recommended for HIV prevention. The vaginal contraceptive sponge, which is not available in the United States, protects against cervical gonorrhea and chlamydia, but its use increases the risk for candidiasis. In case-control and cross-sectional studies, diaphragm use has been demonstrated to protect against cervical gonorrhea, chlamydia, and trichomoniasis; however, no cohort studies have been conducted. Vaginal sponges or diaphragms should not be assumed to protect women against HIV infection. The role of spermicides, sponges, and diaphragms for preventing STDs in men has not been evaluated.

Nonbarrier Contraception, Surgical Sterilization, and Hysterectomy

Women who are not at risk for pregnancy might incorrectly perceive themselves to be at no risk for STDs, including HIV infection. Nonbarrier contraceptive methods offer no protection against HIV or other STDs. Hormonal contraception (e.g., oral contraceptives, Norplant™, and Depo-Provera™) has been associated in some cohort studies with cervical STDs and increased acquisition of HIV; however, data concerning this latter finding are inconsistent. Women who use hormonal contraception, have been surgically sterilized, or have had hysterectomies should be counseled regarding the use of condoms and the risk for STDs, including HIV infection.

HIV Prevention Counseling

Knowledge of HIV status and appropriate counseling are important components in initiating behavior change. Therefore, HIV counseling is an important HIV prevention strategy, although its efficacy in reducing risk behaviors is still being evaluated. By ensuring that counseling is empathic and client-centered, clinicians can develop a realistic appraisal of the patient's risk and help the patient develop a specific and realistic HIV prevention plan (5).

Counseling associated with HIV testing has two main components: pretest and posttest counseling. During pretest counseling, the clinician should conduct a personalized risk assessment, explain the meaning of positive and negative test results, ask for informed consent for the HIV test, and help the patient develop a realistic, personalized risk-reduction plan. During posttest counseling, the clinician should inform the patient of the results, review the meaning of the results, and reinforce prevention messages. If the patient has a confirmed positive HIV test result, posttest counseling should include referral for follow-up medical services and, if needed, social and psychological services. HIV-negative patients at continuing risk for HIV infection also may benefit from referral for additional counseling and prevention services.

Partner Notification

For most STDs, partners of patients should be examined. When exposure to a treatable STD is considered likely, appropriate antimicrobials should be administered even though no clinical signs of infection are evident and laboratory test results are not yet available. In many states, the local or state health department can assist in notifying the partners of patients who have selected STDs (e.g., HIV infection, syphilis, gonorrhea, hepatitis B, and chlamydia).

Health-care providers should advise patients who have an STD to notify sex partners, including those without symptoms, of their exposure and encourage these partners to seek clinical evaluation. This type of partner notification is known as patient referral. In situations in which patient referral may not be effective or possible, health departments should be prepared to assist the patient either through contract referral or provider referral. Contract referral is the process by which patients agree to self-refer their partners within a defined time period. If the partners do not obtain medical evaluation and treatment within that period, then provider referral is implemented. Provider referral is the process by which partners named by infected patients are notified and counseled by health department staff.

Interrupting the transmission of infection is crucial to STD control. For treatable and vaccine-preventable STDs, further transmission and reinfection can be prevented by referral of sex partners for diagnosis, treatment, vaccination (if applicable), and counseling. When health-care providers refer infected patients to local or state health departments for provider-referral partner notification, the patients may be interviewed by trained professionals to obtain the names of their sex partners and information regarding the location of these partners for notification purposes. Every health department protects the privacy of patients in partner-notification activities. Because of the advantage of confidentiality, many patients prefer that public health officials notify partners. However, the ability of public health officials to provide appropriate prophylaxis to contacts of all patients who have STDs may be limited. In situations where the number of anonymous partners is substantial (e.g., situations among persons who exchange sex for drugs), targeted screening of persons at risk may be more effective at stopping the transmission of disease than provider-referral partner notification. Guidelines for management of sex partners and recommendations for partner notification for specific STDs are included for each STD addressed in this report.

Reporting and Confidentiality

The accurate identification and timely reporting of STDs are integral components of successful disease control efforts. Timely reporting is important for assessing morbidity trends, targeting limited resources, and assisting local health authorities in identifying sex partners who may be infected. STD/HIV and acquired immunodeficiency syndrome (AIDS) cases should be reported in accordance with local statutory requirements.

Syphilis, gonorrhea, and AIDS are reportable diseases in every state. Chlamydial infection is reportable in most states. The requirements for reporting other STDs differ by state, and clinicians should be familiar with local STD reporting requirements. Reporting may be provider- and/or laboratory-based. Clinicians who are unsure of local reporting requirements should seek advice from local health departments or state STD programs.

STD and HIV reports are maintained in strictest confidence; in most jurisdictions, such reports are protected by statute from subpoena. Before public health representatives conduct follow-up of a positive STD-test result, these persons should consult the patient's health-care provider to verify the diagnosis and treatment.

SPECIAL POPULATIONS

Pregnant Women

Intrauterine or perinatally transmitted STDs can have fatal or severely debilitating effects on a fetus. Pregnant women and their sex partners should be questioned about STDs and should be counseled about the possibility of perinatal infections.

Recommended Screening Tests

- A serologic test for syphilis should be performed on all pregnant women at the first prenatal visit. In populations in which utilization of prenatal care is not optimal, rapid plasma reagin (RPR)-card test screening and treatment, if that test is reactive, should be performed at the time a pregnancy is diagnosed. For patients at high risk, screening should be repeated in the third trimester and again at delivery. Some states also mandate screening all women at delivery. No infant should be discharged from the hospital without the syphilis serologic status of its mother having been determined at least one time during pregnancy and, preferably, again at delivery. Any woman who delivers a stillborn infant should be tested for syphilis.

- A serologic test for hepatitis B surface antigen (HBsAg) should be performed for all pregnant women at the first prenatal visit. HBsAg testing should be repeated late in the pregnancy for women who are HBsAg negative but who are at high risk for HBV infection (e.g., injecting-drug users and women who have concomitant STDs).

- A test for *Neisseria gonorrhoeae* should be performed at the first prenatal visit for women at risk or for women living in an area in which the prevalence of *N. gonorrhoeae* is high. A repeat test should be performed during the third trimester for those at continued risk.

- A test for *Chlamydia trachomatis* should be performed in the third trimester for women at increased risk (i.e., women aged <25 years and women who have a new or more than one sex partner or whose partner has other partners) to prevent maternal postnatal complications and chlamydial infection in the infant. Screening during the first trimester might enable prevention of adverse effects of chlamydia during pregnancy. However, evidence for adverse effects during pregnancy is minimal. If screening is performed only during the first trimester, a longer period exists for acquiring infection before delivery.

- A test for HIV infection should be offered to all pregnant women at the first prenatal visit.

- A test for bacterial vaginosis (BV) may be conducted early in the second trimester for asymptomatic patients who are at high risk for preterm labor (e.g., those who have a history of a previous preterm delivery). Current evidence does not support universal testing for BV.

- A Papanicolaou (Pap) smear should be obtained at the first prenatal visit if none has been documented during the preceding year.

Other Concerns

Other STD-related concerns are to be considered as follows:

- Pregnant women who have either primary genital herpes infection, HBV, primary cytomegalovirus (CMV) infection, or Group B streptococcal infection and women who have syphilis and who are allergic to penicillin may need to be referred to an expert for management.

- HBsAg-positive pregnant women should be reported to the local and/or state health department to ensure that they are entered into a case-management system and appropriate prophylaxis is provided for their infants. In addition, household and sexual contacts of HBsAg-positive women should be vaccinated.

- In the absence of lesions during the third trimester, routine serial cultures for herpes simplex virus (HSV) are not indicated for women who have a history of recurrent genital herpes. However, obtaining cultures from such women at the time of delivery may be useful in guiding neonatal management. Prophylactic cesarean section is not indicated for women who do not have active genital lesions at the time of delivery.

- The presence of genital warts is not an indication for cesarean section.

For a more detailed discussion of these guidelines, as well as for infections not transmitted sexually, refer to *Guidelines for Perinatal Care* (*6*).

NOTE: The sources for these guidelines for screening of pregnant women include the *Guide to Clinical Preventive Services* (*7*), *Guidelines for Perinatal Care* (*6*), *American College of Obstetricians and Gynecologists (ACOG) Technical Bulletin: Gonorrhea and Chlamydial Infections* (*8*), "Recommendations for the Prevention and Management of *Chlamydia trachomatis* Infections" (*9*), and "Hepatitis B Virus: A Comprehensive Strategy for Eliminating Transmission in the United States through Universal Childhood Vaccination—Recommendations of the Immunization Practices Advisory Committee (ACIP)" (*1*). These sources are not entirely compatible in their recommendations. The *Guide to Clinical Preventive Services* recommends screening of patients at high risk for chlamydia, but indicates that the optimal timing for screening is uncertain. The *Guidelines for Perinatal Care* recommend that pregnant women at high risk for chlamydia be screened for the infection during the first prenatal-care visit and during the third trimester. Recommendations to screen pregnant women for STDs are based on disease severity and sequelae, prevalence in the population, costs, medicolegal considerations (e.g., state laws), and other factors. The screening recommendations in this report are more extensive (i.e., if followed, more women will be screened for more STDs than would be screened by following other recommendations) and are compatible with other CDC guidelines. Physicians should select a screening strategy that is compatible with the population and setting of their medical practices and that meets their goals for STD case detection and treatment.

Adolescents

Health-care providers who provide care for adolescents should be aware of several issues that relate specifically to these persons. The rates of many STDs are highest among adolescents (e.g., the rate of gonorrhea is highest among females aged 15–19 years). Clinic-based studies have demonstrated that the prevalence of chlamydial infections, and possibly of human papillomavirus (HPV) infections, also is highest among adolescents. In addition, surveillance data indicate that 9% of adolescents who have acute HBV infection either a) have had sexual contact with a chronically infected person or with multiple sex partners or b) gave their sexual preference as homosexual. As part of a comprehensive strategy to eliminate HBV transmission in the United States, ACIP has recommended that all children be administered hepatitis B vaccine.

Adolescents who are at high risk for STDs include male homosexuals, sexually active heterosexuals, clients in STD clinics, and injecting-drug users. Younger adolescents (i.e., persons aged <15 years) who are sexually active are at particular risk for infection. Adolescents are at greatest risk for STDs because they frequently have unprotected intercourse, are biologically more susceptible to infection, and face multiple obstacles to utilization of health care.

Several of these issues can be addressed by clinicians who provide services to adolescents. Clinicians can address the general lack of knowledge and awareness about the risks and consequences of STDs and offer guidance, constituting true primary prevention, to help adolescents develop healthy sexual behaviors and prevent the establishment of patterns of behavior that can undermine sexual health. With limited exceptions, all adolescents in the United States can consent to the confidential diagnosis and treatment of STDs. Medical care for STDs can be provided to adolescents without parental consent or knowledge. Furthermore, in many states adolescents can consent to HIV counseling and testing. Consent laws for vaccination of adolescents differ by state. Several states consider provision of vaccine similar to treatment of STDs and provide vaccination services without parental consent. Providers should appreciate how important confidentiality is to adolescents and should strive to follow policies that comply with state laws to ensure the confidentiality of STD-related services provided to adolescents.

The style and content of counseling and health education should be adapted for adolescents. Discussions should be appropriate for the patient's developmental level and should identify risky behaviors, such as sex and drug-use behaviors. Careful counseling and thorough discussions are especially important for adolescents who may not acknowledge engaging in high-risk behaviors. Care and counseling should be direct and nonjudgmental.

Children

Management of children who have STDs requires close cooperation between the clinician, laboratorians, and child-protection authorities. Investigations, when indicated, should be initiated promptly. Some diseases (e.g., gonorrhea, syphilis, and chlamydia), if acquired after the neonatal period, are almost 100% indicative of sexual contact. For other diseases, such as HPV infection and vaginitis, the association with sexual contact is not as clear (see Sexual Assault and STDs).

HIV INFECTION: DETECTION, INITIAL MANAGEMENT, AND REFERRAL

Infection with HIV produces a spectrum of disease that progresses from a clinically latent or asymptomatic state to AIDS as a late manifestation. The pace of disease progression is variable. The time between infection with HIV and the development of AIDS ranges from a few months to as long as 17 years (median: 10 years). Most adults and adolescents infected with HIV remain symptom-free for long periods, but viral replication is active during all stages of infection, increasing substantially as the immune system deteriorates. AIDS eventually develops in almost all HIV-infected persons; in one study of HIV-infected adults, AIDS developed in 87% (95% confidence interval [CI]=83%–90%) within 17 years after infection. Additional cases are expected to occur among those who have remained AIDS-free for longer periods.

Greater awareness among both patients and health-care providers of the risk factors associated with HIV transmission has led to increased testing for HIV and earlier diagnosis of the infection, often before symptoms develop. The early diagnosis of HIV infection is important for several reasons. Treatments are available to slow the decline of immune system function. HIV-infected persons who have altered immune function are at increased risk for infections for which preventive measures are available (e.g., *Pneumocystis carinii* pneumonia [PCP], toxoplasmic encephalitis [TE], disseminated *Mycobacterium avium* complex [MAC] disease, tuberculosis [TB], and bacterial pneumonia). Because of its effect on the immune system, HIV affects the diagnosis, evaluation, treatment, and follow-up of many other diseases and may affect the efficacy of antimicrobial therapy for some STDs. Finally, the early diagnosis of HIV enables the health-care provider to counsel such patients and to assist in preventing HIV transmission to others.

Proper management of HIV infection involves a complex array of behavioral, psychosocial, and medical services. Although some of these services may be available in the STD treatment facility, other services, particularly medical services, are usually unavailable in this setting. Therefore, referral to a health-care provider or facility experienced in caring for HIV-infected patients is advised. Staff in STD treatment facilities should be knowledgeable about the options for referral available in their communities. While in the STD treatment facility, the HIV-infected patient should be educated about HIV infection and the various options for HIV care that are available.

Because of the complexity of services required for management of HIV infection, detailed information, particularly regarding medical care, is beyond the scope of this report and may be found elsewhere (*3,5,10,11*). Rather, this section provides information on diagnostic testing for HIV-1 and HIV-2, counseling patients who have HIV infection, and preparing the HIV-infected patient for what to expect when medical care is necessary. Information also is provided on management of sex partners, because such services can and should be provided in the STD treatment facility before referral. Finally, the topics of HIV infection during pregnancy and in infants and children are addressed.

Diagnostic Testing for HIV-1 and HIV-2

Testing for HIV should be offered to all persons whose behavior puts them at risk for infection, including persons who seek evaluation and treatment for STDs. Counseling before and after testing (i.e., pretest and posttest counseling) is an integral part of the testing procedure (see HIV Prevention Counseling). Informed consent must be obtained before an HIV test is performed. Some states require written consent.

HIV infection usually is diagnosed by using HIV-1 antibody tests. Antibody testing begins with a sensitive screening test such as the enzyme immunoassay (EIA). Reactive screening tests must be confirmed by a supplemental test, such as the Western blot (WB) or an immunofluorescence assay (IFA). If confirmed by a supplemental test, a positive antibody test result indicates that a person is infected with HIV and is capable of transmitting the virus to others. HIV antibody is detectable in at least 95% of patients within 6 months after infection. Although a negative antibody test result usually indicates that a person is not infected, antibody tests cannot exclude infection that occurred <6 months before the test.

The prevalence of HIV-2 in the United States is extremely low, and CDC does not recommend routine testing for HIV-2 in settings other than blood centers, unless demographic or behavioral information indicates that HIV-2 infection might be present. Those at risk for HIV-2 infection include persons from a country in which HIV-2 is endemic or the sex partners of such persons. HIV-2 is endemic in parts of West Africa, and an increased prevalence of HIV-2 has been reported in Angola, France, Mozambique, and Portugal. In addition, testing for HIV-2 should be conducted when there is clinical evidence or suspicion of HIV disease in the absence of a positive test for antibodies to HIV-1 (*12*).

Because HIV antibody crosses the placenta, its presence in a child aged <18 months is not diagnostic of HIV infection (see Special Considerations, HIV Infection in Infants and Children).

The following are specific recommendations for diagnostic testing for HIV infection:

• Informed consent must be obtained before an HIV test is performed. Some states require written consent. (See HIV Prevention Counseling for a discussion of pretest and posttest counseling.)

- Positive screening tests for HIV antibody must be confirmed by a more specific confirmatory test (either WB or IFA) before being considered diagnostic of HIV infection.

- Patients who have positive HIV test results must either receive behavioral, psychosocial, and medical evaluation and monitoring services or be referred for these services.

Acute Retroviral Syndrome

Health-care providers should be alert for the symptoms and signs of acute retroviral syndrome, which is characterized by fever, malaise, lymphadenopathy, and skin rash. This syndrome frequently occurs in the first few weeks after HIV infection, before antibody test results become positive. Suspicion of acute retroviral syndrome should prompt nucleic acid testing to detect the presence of HIV. Recent data indicate that initiation of antiretroviral therapy during this period can delay the onset of HIV-related complications and might influence prognosis. If testing reveals acute HIV infection, health-care providers should either counsel the patient about immediate initiation of antiretroviral therapy or refer the patient for emergency expert consultation. The optimal antiretroviral regimen at this time is unknown. Treatment with zidovudine can delay the onset of HIV-related complications; however, most experts recommend treatment with two nucleoside reverse transcriptase inhibitors and a protease inhibitor.

Counseling for HIV-Infected Patients

Behavioral and psychosocial services are an integral part of health care for HIV-infected patients; such services should be available on-site or through referral when HIV infection is diagnosed. Patients often are distressed when first informed of a positive HIV test result. Such patients face several major adaptive challenges: a) accepting the possibility of a shortened life span, b) coping with others' reactions to a stigmatizing illness, c) developing and adopting strategies for maintaining physical and emotional health, and d) initiating changes in behavior to prevent HIV transmission to others. Many patients also require assistance with making reproductive choices, gaining access to health services, and confronting employment or housing discrimination.

Interrupting HIV transmission depends on behavioral changes made by those persons at risk for transmitting or acquiring infection. Infected persons, as potential sources of new infections, must receive additional counseling and assistance to support partner notification and counseling to prevent infection of others. Targeting behavior change programs toward HIV-infected persons and their sex partners, or those with whom they share injecting-drug equipment, is an important adjunct to AIDS prevention efforts.

The following are specific recommendations for counseling HIV-infected patients:

- Persons who test positive for HIV antibody should be counseled by a person or persons, either on-site or through referral, who can discuss the behavioral, psychosocial, and medical implications of HIV infection.

- Appropriate social support and psychological resources should be available, either on-site or through referral, to assist patients in coping with emotional distress.

- Persons who continue to be at risk for transmitting HIV should receive assistance in changing or avoiding behaviors that can transmit infection to others.

Planning for Medical Care and for Continuation of Psychosocial Services

Practice settings for offering HIV care differ depending on local resources and needs. Primary-care providers and outpatient facilities must ensure that appropriate resources are available for each patient and must avoid fragmentation of care as much as possible. A single source that is able to provide comprehensive care for all stages of HIV infection is preferred; however, the limited availability of such resources often results in the need to coordinate care among outpatient, inpatient, and specialist providers in different locations. Providers should do everything possible to avoid fragmentation of care and long delays between diagnosis of HIV infection and access to medical and psychosocial services.

Recently identified HIV infection may not have been recently acquired. Persons newly diagnosed with HIV may be at any of the different stages of infection. Therefore, the health-care provider should be alert for symptoms or signs that suggest advanced HIV infection (e.g., fever, weight loss, diarrhea, cough, shortness of breath, and oral candidiasis). The presence of any of these symptoms should prompt urgent referral for medical care. Similarly, the provider should be alert for signs of severe psychologic distress and be prepared to refer the client accordingly.

HIV-infected patients in the STD treatment setting should be educated about what to expect when medical care is necessary (11). In the nonemergent situation, the initial evaluation of the HIV-positive patient usually includes the following components:

- A detailed medical history, including sexual and substance-abuse history, previous STDs, and specific HIV-related symptoms or diagnoses.

- A physical examination; for women, this should include a gynecologic examination.

- For women, testing for *N. gonorrhoeae* and *C. trachomatis*, a Pap smear, and wet mount examination of vaginal secretions.

- Complete blood and platelet counts and blood chemistry profile.

- Toxoplasma antibody test, tests for hepatitis B viral markers, and syphilis serology.

- A CD4+ T-lymphocyte analysis and determination of HIV plasma ribonucleic acid (i.e., HIV viral load).

- A tuberculin skin test (TST) (sometimes referred to as a purified protein derivative [PPD] skin test) administered by the Mantoux method. The test result should be evaluated at 48–72 hours; in HIV-infected persons, a 5 mm induration is considered positive. The usefulness of anergy testing is controversial (*13–15*).

- A chest radiograph.

- A thorough psychosocial evaluation, including ascertainment of behavioral factors indicating risk for transmitting HIV and elucidation of information concerning any partners who should be notified about possible exposure to HIV.

In subsequent visits, once the results of laboratory and skin tests are available, the patient may be offered antiretroviral therapy (*16*), as well as specific medications to reduce the incidence of opportunistic infections (e.g., PCP, TE, disseminated MAC infection, and TB) (*10,14,17–19*). Hepatitis B vaccination should be offered to patients who do not have hepatitis B markers, influenza vaccination should be offered annually, and pneumococcal vaccination should be administered. For additional information concerning vaccination of HIV-infected patients, refer to "Recommendations of the Advisory Committee on Immunization Practices (ACIP): Use of Vaccines and Immune Globulins in Persons with Altered Immunocompetence" (*20*).

Specific recommendations for planning medical care and continuation of psychosocial services include the following:

- HIV-infected persons should be referred for appropriate follow-up to facilities in which health-care personnel are experienced in providing care for HIV-infected patients.

- Health-care providers should be alert for medical or psychosocial conditions that require immediate attention.

- Patients should be educated about what to expect in follow-up medical care.

Management of Sex Partners and Injecting-Drug Partners

When referring to persons who are infected with HIV, the term "partner" includes not only sex partners but also injecting-drug users who share syringes or other injection equipment. The rationale for partner notification is that the early diagnosis and treatment of HIV infection possibly reduces morbidity and provides the opportunity to encourage risk-reducing behaviors. Partner notification for HIV infection must be confidential and will depend on voluntary cooperation of the patient.

Two complementary notification processes, patient referral and provider referral, can be used to identify partners. With patient referral, patients directly inform their partners of their exposure to HIV infection. With provider referral, trained health department personnel locate partners on the basis of the names, descriptions, and addresses provided by the patient. During the notification process, the anonymity of patients is protected; their names are not revealed to partners who are notified. Many state health departments provide assistance, if requested, with provider-referral partner notification.

The results of one randomized trial suggested that provider referral is more effective in notifying partners than patient referral. In that study, 50% of partners in the provider-referral group were notified, compared with 7% of partners notified by persons in the patient-referral group. However, whether behavioral change takes place as a result of partner notification has not been determined, and many patients are reluctant to disclose the names of partners because of concern about discrimination, disruption of relationships, loss of confidentiality for the partners, and possible violence.

The following are specific recommendations for implementing partner-notification procedures:

- HIV-infected patients should be encouraged to notify their partners and to refer them for counseling and testing. If requested by the patient, health-care providers should assist in this process, either directly or by referral to health department partner-notification programs.

- If patients are unwilling to notify their partners, or if they cannot ensure that their partners will seek counseling, physicians or health department personnel should use confidential procedures to notify the partners.

Special Considerations

Pregnancy

All pregnant women should be offered HIV testing as early in pregnancy as possible (21). This recommendation is particularly important because of the available treatments for reducing the likelihood of perinatal transmission and maintaining the health of the woman. HIV-infected women should be informed specifically about the risk for perinatal infection. Current evidence indicates that 15%–25% of infants born to untreated HIV-infected mothers are infected with HIV; the virus also can be transmitted from an infected mother by breastfeeding. Zidovudine (ZDV) reduces the risk for HIV transmission to the infant from approximately 25% to 8% if administered to women during the later stage of pregnancy and during labor and to infants for the first 6 weeks of life (22). Therefore, ZDV treatment should be offered to all HIV-infected pregnant women. In the United States, HIV-infected women should be advised not to breastfeed their infants.

Insufficient information is available regarding the safety of ZDV or other antiretroviral drugs during early pregnancy; however, on the basis of the ACTG-076
protocol,* ZDV is indicated for the prevention of maternal-fetal HIV transmission as
part of a regimen that includes oral ZDV at 14–34 weeks of gestation, intravenous
(IV) ZDV during labor, and ZDV Syrup to the neonate after birth (22). Glaxo Well-
come, Inc., Hoffmann-LaRoche, Inc., Bristol-Myers Squibb, Co., and Merck & Co.,
Inc., in cooperation with CDC, maintain a registry to assess the safety of ZDV,
didanosine (ddI), lamivudine (3TC), saquinavir (SAQ), stavudine (d4t), and dideoxy-
cytodine (ddC) during pregnancy. Women who receive any of these drugs during
pregnancy should be reported to this registry; telephone (800) 722-9292, extension
38465. The number of cases reported through February 1997 represented a sample
of insufficient size for reliably estimating the risk for birth defects after administration of ddI, 3TC, SAQ, d4t, ddC, or ZDV, or their combination, to pregnant women
and their fetuses. However, the registry findings did not indicate an increase in the
number of birth defects after receipt of only ZDV in comparison with the number
expected in the U.S. population. Furthermore, no consistent pattern of birth defects
has been observed that would suggest a common cause.

Women should be counseled about their options regarding pregnancy. The objective of counseling is to provide HIV-infected women with information for making
reproductive decisions, analogous to the model used in genetic counseling. In addition, contraceptive counseling should be offered to HIV-infected women who do
not desire pregnancy. Prenatal and abortion services should be available on-site or
by referral. Pregnancy among HIV-infected women does not appear to increase maternal morbidity or mortality.

HIV Infection in Infants and Children

HIV-infected infants and young children differ from adults and adolescents with
respect to the diagnosis, clinical presentation, and management of HIV disease. For
example, because of transplacental passage of maternal HIV antibody, both infected and uninfected infants born to HIV-infected mothers are expected to have
positive HIV-antibody test results. A definitive determination of HIV infection in a
child <18 months of age should be based on laboratory evidence of HIV in blood or
tissues by culture, nucleic acid, or antigen detection. In addition, CD4+ lymphocyte
counts are higher in infants and children aged <5 years than in healthy adults and
must be interpreted accordingly. All infants born to HIV-infected mothers should
begin PCP prophylaxis at age 4–6 weeks; such prophylaxis should be continued
until HIV infection has been excluded (18). Other modifications must be made in
health services that are recommended for infants and children, such as avoiding
vaccination with live oral polio vaccine when a child (or household contact) is infected with HIV. Management of infants, children, and adolescents who are known
or suspected to be infected with HIV requires referral to physicians familiar with the
manifestations and treatment of pediatric HIV infection.

---

*The Acquired Immunodeficiency Syndrome (AIDS) Clinical Trials Group Protocol 076, a clinical
trial sponsored by the National Institutes of Health in collaboration with the National Institute
of Health and Medical Research and the National Agency of Research on AIDS in France.

DISEASES CHARACTERIZED BY GENITAL ULCERS

Management of Patients Who Have Genital Ulcers

In the United States, most young, sexually active patients who have genital ulcers have either genital herpes, syphilis, or chancroid. The relative frequency of each differs by geographic area and patient population; however, in most areas of the United States, genital herpes is the most prevalent of these diseases. More than one of these diseases could be present in a patient who has genital ulcers. Each disease has been associated with an increased risk for HIV infection.

A diagnosis based only on the patient's medical history and physical examination often is inaccurate. Therefore, evaluation of all patients who have genital ulcers should include a serologic test for syphilis and diagnostic evaluation for herpes. Although, ideally, all of these tests should be conducted for each patient who has a genital ulcer, use of such tests (other than a serologic test for syphilis) may be based on test availability and clinical or epidemiologic suspicion. Specific tests for the evaluation of genital ulcers include the following:

- Darkfield examination or direct immunofluorescence test for *Treponema pallidum*,

- Culture or antigen test for HSV, and

- Culture for *Haemophilus ducreyi*.

Polymerase chain reaction (PCR) tests for these organisms might become available commercially.

HIV testing should be a) performed in the management of patients who have genital ulcers caused by *T. pallidum* or *H. ducreyi* and b) considered for those who have ulcers caused by HSV (see sections on Syphilis, Chancroid, and Genital Herpes).

A health-care provider often must treat a patient before test results are available. In such a circumstance, the clinician should treat for the diagnosis considered most likely. If the diagnosis is unclear, many experts recommend treatment for syphilis, or for both syphilis and chancroid if the patient resides in a community in which *H. ducreyi* is a significant cause of genital ulcers, especially when diagnostic capabilities for chancroid or syphilis are not ideal. However, even after complete diagnostic evaluation, at least 25% of patients who have genital ulcers have no laboratory-confirmed diagnosis.

Chancroid

Chancroid is endemic in some areas of the United States, and the disease also occurs in discrete outbreaks. Chancroid is a cofactor for HIV transmission, and high rates of HIV infection among patients who have chancroid have been reported in the United States and other countries. An estimated 10% of patients who have chancroid could be coinfected with *T. pallidum* or HSV.

A definitive diagnosis of chancroid requires identification of *H. ducreyi* on special culture media that are not widely available from commercial sources; even using these media, sensitivity is ≤80%. A probable diagnosis, for both clinical and surveillance purposes, may be made if the following criteria are met: a) the patient has one or more painful genital ulcers; b) the patient has no evidence of *T. pallidum* infection by darkfield examination of ulcer exudate or by a serologic test for syphilis performed at least 7 days after onset of ulcers; and c) the clinical presentation, appearance of genital ulcers, and regional lymphadenopathy, if present, are typical for chancroid and a test for HSV is negative. The combination of a painful ulcer and tender inguinal adenopathy, which occurs among one third of patients, suggests a diagnosis of chancroid; when accompanied by suppurative inguinal adenopathy, these signs are almost pathognomonic. PCR testing for *H. ducreyi* might become available soon.

Treatment

Successful treatment for chancroid cures the infection, resolves the clinical symptoms, and prevents transmission to others. In extensive cases, scarring can result despite successful therapy.

Recommended Regimens

Azithromycin 1 g orally in a single dose,
OR
Ceftriaxone 250 mg intramuscularly (IM) in a single dose,
OR
Ciprofloxacin 500 mg orally twice a day for 3 days,
OR
Erythromycin base 500 mg orally four times a day for 7 days.

NOTE: Ciprofloxacin is contraindicated for pregnant and lactating women and for persons aged <18 years.

All four regimens are effective for treatment of chancroid in HIV-infected patients. Azithromycin and ceftriaxone offer the advantage of single-dose therapy. Worldwide, several isolates with intermediate resistance to either ciprofloxacin or erythromycin have been reported.

Other Management Considerations

Patients who are uncircumcised and HIV-infected patients might not respond as well to treatment as those who are circumcised or HIV-negative. Patients should be tested for HIV infection at the time chancroid is diagnosed. Patients should be retested 3 months after the diagnosis of chancroid if the initial test results for syphilis and HIV were negative.

Follow-Up

Patients should be reexamined 3–7 days after initiation of therapy. If treatment is successful, ulcers improve symptomatically within 3 days and objectively within

7 days after therapy. If no clinical improvement is evident, the clinician must consider whether a) the diagnosis is correct, b) the patient is coinfected with another STD, c) the patient is infected with HIV, d) the treatment was not taken as instructed, or e) the *H. ducreyi* strain causing the infection is resistant to the prescribed antimicrobial. The time required for complete healing depends on the size of the ulcer; large ulcers may require >2 weeks. In addition, healing is slower for some uncircumcised men who have ulcers under the foreskin. Clinical resolution of fluctuant lymphadenopathy is slower than that of ulcers and may require drainage, even during otherwise successful therapy. Although needle aspiration of buboes is a simpler procedure, incision and drainage of buboes may be preferred because of less need for subsequent drainage procedures.

Management of Sex Partners

Sex partners of patients who have chancroid should be examined and treated, regardless of whether symptoms of the disease are present, if they had sexual contact with the patient during the 10 days preceding onset of symptoms in the patient.

Special Considerations

Pregnancy

The safety of azithromycin for pregnant and lactating women has not been established. Ciprofloxacin is contraindicated during pregnancy. No adverse effects of chancroid on pregnancy outcome or on the fetus have been reported.

HIV Infection

HIV-infected patients who have chancroid should be monitored closely. Such patients may require longer courses of therapy than those recommended for HIV-negative patients. Healing may be slower among HIV-infected patients, and treatment failures occur with any regimen. Because data are limited concerning the therapeutic efficacy of the recommended ceftriaxone and azithromycin regimens in HIV-infected patients, these regimens should be used for such patients only if follow-up can be ensured. Some experts suggest using the erythromycin 7-day regimen for treating HIV-infected persons.

Genital Herpes Simplex Virus (HSV) Infection

Genital herpes is a recurrent, incurable viral disease. Two serotypes of HSV have been identified: HSV-1 and HSV-2. Most cases of recurrent genital herpes are caused by HSV-2. On the basis of serologic studies, genital HSV-2 infection has been diagnosed in at least 45 million persons in the United States.

Most HSV-2–infected persons have not received a diagnosis of genital herpes. Such persons have mild or unrecognized infections that shed virus intermittently in the genital tract. Some cases of first-episode genital herpes are manifested by severe disease that might require hospitalization. Many cases of genital herpes are transmitted by persons who are unaware that they have the infection or are asymptomatic when transmission occurs.

Systemic antiviral drugs partially control the symptoms and signs of herpes episodes when used to treat first clinical episodes or recurrent episodes or when used as daily suppressive therapy. However, these drugs neither eradicate latent virus nor affect the risk, frequency, or severity of recurrences after the drug is discontinued. Randomized trials indicate that three antiviral medications provide clinical benefit for genital herpes: acyclovir, valacyclovir, and famciclovir. Valacyclovir is a valine ester of acyclovir with enhanced absorption after oral administration. Famciclovir, a prodrug of penciclovir, also has high oral bioavailability. Topical therapy with acyclovir is substantially less effective than the systemic drug, and its use is discouraged. The recommended acyclovir dosing regimens for both initial and recurrent episodes reflect substantial clinical experience, expert opinion, and FDA-approved dosages.

First Clinical Episode of Genital Herpes

Management of patients with first clinical episode of genital herpes includes antiviral therapy and counseling regarding the natural history of genital herpes, sexual and perinatal transmission, and methods to reduce such transmission. Five percent to 30% of first-episode cases of genital herpes are caused by HSV-1, but clinical recurrences are much less frequent for HSV-1 than HSV-2 genital infection. Therefore, identification of the type of the infecting strain has prognostic importance and may be useful for counseling purposes.

Recommended Regimens

Acyclovir 400 mg orally three times a day for 7–10 days,
OR
Acyclovir 200 mg orally five times a day for 7–10 days,
OR
Famciclovir 250 mg orally three times a day for 7–10 days,
OR
Valacyclovir 1 g orally twice a day for 7–10 days.

NOTE: Treatment may be extended if healing is incomplete after 10 days of therapy.

Higher dosages of acyclovir (i.e., 400 mg orally five times a day) were used in treatment studies of first-episode herpes proctitis and first-episode oral infection, including stomatitis or pharyngitis. It is unclear whether these forms of mucosal infection require higher doses of acyclovir than used for genital herpes. Valacyclovir and famciclovir probably are also effective for acute HSV proctitis or oral infection, but clinical experience is lacking.

Counseling is an important aspect of managing patients who have genital herpes. Although initial counseling can be provided at the first visit, many patients benefit from learning about the chronic aspects of the disease after the acute illness subsides. Counseling of these patients should include the following:

● Patients who have genital herpes should be told about the natural history of the disease, with emphasis on the potential for recurrent episodes, asymptomatic viral shedding, and sexual transmission.

- Patients should be advised to abstain from sexual activity when lesions or prodromal symptoms are present and encouraged to inform their sex partners that they have genital herpes. The use of condoms during all sexual exposures with new or uninfected sex partners should be encouraged.

- Sexual transmission of HSV can occur during asymptomatic periods. Asymptomatic viral shedding occurs more frequently in patients who have genital HSV-2 infection than HSV-1 infection and in patients who have had genital herpes for <12 months. Such patients should be counseled to prevent spread of the infection.

- The risk for neonatal infection should be explained to all patients, including men. Childbearing-aged women who have genital herpes should be advised to inform health-care providers who care for them during pregnancy about the HSV infection.

- Patients having a first episode of genital herpes should be advised that a) episodic antiviral therapy during recurrent episodes might shorten the duration of lesions and b) suppressive antiviral therapy can ameliorate or prevent recurrent outbreaks.

Recurrent Episodes of HSV Disease

Most patients with first-episode genital HSV-2 infection will have recurrent episodes of genital lesions. Episodic or suppressive antiviral therapy might shorten the duration of lesions or ameliorate recurrences. Because many patients benefit from antiviral therapy, options for treatment should be discussed with all patients.

When treatment is started during the prodrome or within 1 day after onset of lesions, many patients who have recurrent disease benefit from episodic therapy. If episodic treatment of recurrences is chosen, the patient should be provided with antiviral therapy, or a prescription for the medication, so that treatment can be initiated at the first sign of prodrome or genital lesions.

Daily suppressive therapy reduces the frequency of genital herpes recurrences by ≥75% among patients who have frequent recurrences (i.e., six or more recurrences per year). Safety and efficacy have been documented among patients receiving daily therapy with acyclovir for as long as 6 years, and with valacyclovir and famciclovir for 1 year. Suppressive therapy has not been associated with emergence of clinically significant acyclovir resistance among immunocompetent patients. After 1 year of continuous suppressive therapy, discontinuation of therapy should be discussed with the patient to assess the patient's psychological adjustment to genital herpes and rate of recurrent episodes, as the frequency of recurrences decreases over time in many patients. Insufficient experience with famciclovir and valacyclovir prevents recommendation of these drugs for >1 year.

Suppressive treatment with acyclovir reduces but does not eliminate asymptomatic viral shedding. Therefore, the extent to which suppressive therapy may prevent HSV transmission is unknown.

Recommended Regimens for Episodic Recurrent Infection

Acyclovir 400 mg orally three times a day for 5 days,
OR
Acyclovir 200 mg orally five times a day for 5 days,
OR
Acyclovir 800 mg orally twice a day for 5 days,
OR
Famciclovir 125 mg orally twice a day for 5 days,
OR
Valacyclovir 500 mg orally twice a day for 5 days.

Recommended Regimens for Daily Suppressive Therapy

Acyclovir 400 mg orally twice a day,
OR
Famciclovir 250 mg orally twice a day,
OR
Valacyclovir 250 mg orally twice a day,
OR
Valacyclovir 500 mg orally once a day,
OR
Valacyclovir 1,000 mg orally once a day.

Valacyclovir 500 mg once a day appears less effective than other valacyclovir dosing regimens in patients who have very frequent recurrences (i.e., ≥10 episodes per year). Few comparative studies of valacyclovir and famciclovir with acyclovir have been conducted. The results of these studies suggest that valacyclovir and famciclovir are comparable to acyclovir in clinical outcome. However, valacyclovir and famciclovir may provide increased ease in administration, which is an important consideration for prolonged treatment.

Severe Disease

IV therapy should be provided for patients who have severe disease or complications necessitating hospitalization, such as disseminated infection, pneumonitis, hepatitis, or complications of the central nervous system (e.g., meningitis or encephalitis).

Recommended Regimen

Acyclovir 5–10 mg/kg body weight IV every 8 hours for 5–7 days or until clinical resolution is attained.

Management of Sex Partners

The sex partners of patients who have genital herpes are likely to benefit from evaluation and counseling. Symptomatic sex partners should be evaluated and treated in the same manner as patients who have genital lesions. However, most persons who have genital HSV infection do not have a history of typical genital lesions. These persons and their future sex partners may benefit from evaluation and counseling. Thus, even asymptomatic sex partners of patients who have newly diagnosed genital herpes should be questioned concerning histories of typical and atypical genital lesions, and they should be encouraged to examine themselves for lesions in the future and seek medical attention promptly if lesions appear.

Most of the available HSV antibody tests do not accurately discriminate between HSV-1 and HSV-2 antibodies, and their use is not currently recommended. Sensitive and type-specific serum antibody assays may become commercially available and contribute to future intervention strategies.

Special Considerations

Allergy, Intolerance, or Adverse Reactions

Allergic and other adverse reactions to acyclovir, valacyclovir, and famciclovir are infrequent. Desensitization to acyclovir has been described previously (*23*).

HIV Infection

Immunocompromised patients might have prolonged and/or severe episodes of genital or perianal herpes. Lesions caused by HSV are relatively common among HIV-infected patients and may be severe, painful, and atypical. Intermittent or suppressive therapy with oral antiviral agents is often beneficial.

The dosage of antiviral drugs for HIV-infected patients is controversial, but clinical experience strongly suggests that immunocompromised patients benefit from increased doses of antiviral drugs. Regimens such as acyclovir 400 mg orally three to five times a day, as used for other immunocompromised patients, have been useful. Therapy should be continued until clinical resolution is attained. Famciclovir 500 mg twice a day has been effective in decreasing both the rate of recurrences and the rate of subclinical shedding among HIV-infected patients. In immunocompromised patients, valacyclovir in doses of 8 g per day has been associated with a syndrome resembling either hemolytic uremic syndrome or thrombotic thrombocytopenic purpura. However, in the doses recommended for treatment of genital herpes, valacyclovir, acyclovir, and famciclovir probably are safe for use in immunocompromised patients. For severe cases, acyclovir 5 mg/kg IV every 8 hours may be required.

If lesions persist in a patient receiving acyclovir treatment, resistance of the HSV strain to acyclovir should be suspected. Such patients should be managed in consultation with an expert. For severe cases caused by proven or suspected acyclovir-resistant strains, alternate therapy should be administered. All acyclovir-resistant strains are resistant to valacyclovir, and most are resistant to famciclovir. Foscarnet, 40 mg/kg body weight IV every 8 hours until clinical resolution is attained, is often effective for treatment of acyclovir-resistant genital herpes. Topical cidofovir gel 1% applied to the lesions once daily for 5 consecutive days also might be effective.

Pregnancy

The safety of systemic acyclovir and valacyclovir therapy in pregnant women has not been established. Glaxo-Wellcome, Inc., in cooperation with CDC, maintains a registry to assess the use and effects of acyclovir and valacyclovir during pregnancy. Women who receive acyclovir or valacyclovir during pregnancy should be reported to this registry; telephone (800) 722-9292, extension 38465.

Current registry findings do not indicate an increased risk for major birth defects after acyclovir treatment (i.e., in comparison with the general population). These findings provide some assurance in counseling women who have had prenatal exposure to acyclovir. The accumulated case histories represent an insufficient sample for reaching reliable and definitive conclusions regarding the risks associated with acyclovir treatment during pregnancy. Prenatal exposure to valacyclovir and famciclovir is too limited to provide useful information on pregnancy outcomes.

The first clinical episode of genital herpes during pregnancy may be treated with oral acyclovir. In the presence of life-threatening maternal HSV infection (e.g., disseminated infection, encephalitis, pneumonitis, or hepatitis), acyclovir administered IV is indicated. Investigations of acyclovir use among pregnant women suggest that acyclovir treatment near term might reduce the rate of abdominal deliveries among women who have frequently recurring or newly acquired genital herpes by decreasing the incidence of active lesions. However, routine administration of acyclovir to pregnant women who have a history of recurrent genital herpes is not recommended at this time.

Perinatal Infection

Most mothers of infants who acquire neonatal herpes lack histories of clinically evident genital herpes. The risk for transmission to the neonate from an infected mother is high among women who acquire genital herpes near the time of delivery (30%–50%) and is low among women who have a history of recurrent herpes at term and women who acquire genital HSV during the first half of pregnancy (3%). Therefore, prevention of neonatal herpes should emphasize prevention of acquisition of genital HSV infection during late pregnancy. Susceptible women whose partners have oral or genital HSV infection, or those whose sex partners' infection status is unknown, should be counseled to avoid unprotected genital and oral sexual contact during late pregnancy. The results of viral cultures during pregnancy do not predict viral shedding at the time of delivery, and such cultures are not indicated routinely.

At the onset of labor, all women should be examined and carefully questioned regarding whether they have symptoms of genital herpes. Infants of women who do not have symptoms or signs of genital herpes infection or its prodrome may be delivered vaginally. Abdominal delivery does not completely eliminate the risk for HSV infection in the neonate.

Infants exposed to HSV during birth, as proven by virus isolation or presumed by observation of lesions, should be followed carefully. Some authorities recommend that such infants undergo surveillance cultures of mucosal surfaces to detect HSV infection before development of clinical signs. Available data do not support the routine use of acyclovir for asymptomatic infants exposed during birth through an infected birth canal, because the risk for infection in most infants is low. However, infants born to women who acquired genital herpes near term are at high risk for neonatal herpes, and some experts recommend acyclovir therapy for these infants. Such pregnancies and newborns should be managed in consultation with an expert. All infants who have evidence of neonatal herpes should be promptly evaluated and treated with systemic acyclovir (*19*). Acyclovir 30–60 mg/kg/day for 10–21 days is the regimen of choice.

Granuloma Inguinale (Donovanosis)

Granuloma inguinale, a rare disease in the United States, is caused by the intracellular Gram-negative bacterium *Calymmatobacterium granulomatis*. The disease is endemic in certain tropical and developing areas, including India, Papua New Guinea, central Australia, and southern Africa. The disease presents clinically as painless, progressive, ulcerative lesions without regional lymphadenopathy. The lesions are highly vascular (i.e., a beefy red appearance) and bleed easily on contact. The causative organism cannot be cultured on standard microbiologic media, and diagnosis requires visualization of dark-staining Donovan bodies on tissue crush preparation or biopsy. A secondary bacterial infection might develop in the lesions, or the lesions might be coinfected with another sexually transmitted pathogen.

Treatment

Treatment appears to halt progressive destruction of tissue, although prolonged duration of therapy often is required to enable granulation and re-epithelialization of the ulcers. Relapse can occur 6–18 months later despite effective initial therapy.

Recommended Regimens

Trimethoprim-sulfamethoxazole one double-strength tablet orally twice a day for a minimum of 3 weeks,

OR

Doxycycline 100 mg orally twice a day for a minimum of 3 weeks.

Therapy should be continued until all lesions have healed completely.

Alternative Regimens

Ciprofloxacin 750 mg orally twice a day for a minimum of 3 weeks,

OR

Erythromycin base 500 mg orally four times a day for a minimum of 3 weeks.

For any of the above regimens, the addition of an aminoglycoside (gentamicin 1 mg/kg IV every 8 hours) should be considered if lesions do not respond within the first few days of therapy.

Follow-Up

Patients should be followed clinically until signs and symptoms have resolved.

Management of Sex Partners

Sex partners of patients who have granuloma inguinale should be examined and treated if they a) had sexual contact with the patient during the 60 days preceding the onset of symptoms in the patient and b) have clinical signs and symptoms of the disease.

Special Considerations

Pregnancy

Pregnancy is a relative contraindication to the use of sulfonamides. Both pregnant and lactating women should be treated with the erythromycin regimen. The addition of a parenteral aminoglycoside (e.g., gentamicin) should be strongly considered.

HIV Infection

HIV-infected persons who have granuloma inguinale should be treated following the regimens cited previously. The addition of a parenteral aminoglycoside (e.g., gentamicin) should be strongly considered.

Lymphogranuloma Venereum

Lymphogranuloma venereum (LGV), a rare disease in the United States, is caused by the invasive serovars L1, L2, or L3 of *C. trachomatis*. The most frequent clinical manifestation of LGV among heterosexual men is tender inguinal and/or femoral lymphadenopathy that is usually unilateral. Women and homosexually active men might have proctocolitis or inflammatory involvement of perirectal or perianal lymphatic tissues that can result in fistulas and strictures. When most patients seek medical care, they no longer have the self-limited genital ulcer that sometimes occurs at the inoculation site. The diagnosis usually is made serologically and by exclusion of other causes of inguinal lymphadenopathy or genital ulcers.

Treatment

Treatment cures infection and prevents ongoing tissue damage, although tissue reaction can result in scarring. Buboes may require aspiration through intact skin or incision and drainage to prevent the formation of inguinal/femoral ulcerations. Doxycycline is the preferred treatment.

Recommended Regimen

Doxycycline 100 mg orally twice a day for 21 days.

Alternative Regimen

Erythromycin base 500 mg orally four times a day for 21 days.

The activity of azithromycin against *C. trachomatis* suggests that it may be effective in multiple doses over 2–3 weeks, but clinical data regarding its use are lacking.

Follow-Up

Patients should be followed clinically until signs and symptoms have resolved.

Management of Sex Partners

Sex partners of patients who have LGV should be examined, tested for urethral or cervical chlamydial infection, and treated if they had sexual contact with the patient during the 30 days preceding onset of symptoms in the patient.

Special Considerations

Pregnancy

Pregnant women should be treated with the erythromycin regimen.

HIV Infection

HIV-infected persons who have LGV should be treated according to the regimens cited previously. Anecdotal evidence suggests that LGV infection in HIV-positive patients may require prolonged therapy and that resolution might be delayed.

Syphilis

General Principles

Background

Syphilis is a systemic disease caused by *T. pallidum*. Patients who have syphilis may seek treatment for signs or symptoms of primary infection (i.e., ulcer or chancre at the infection site), secondary infection (i.e., manifestations that include rash, mucocutaneous lesions, and adenopathy), or tertiary infection (i.e., cardiac, neurologic, ophthalmic, auditory, or gummatous lesions). Infections also may be detected by serologic testing during the latent stage. Latent syphilis acquired within the preceding year is referred to as early latent syphilis; all other cases of latent syphilis are either late latent syphilis or syphilis of unknown duration. Treatment for late latent syphilis, as well as tertiary syphilis, theoretically may require a longer duration of therapy because organisms are dividing more slowly; however, the validity and importance of this concept have not been determined.

Diagnostic Considerations and Use of Serologic Tests

Darkfield examinations and direct fluorescent antibody tests of lesion exudate or tissue are the definitive methods for diagnosing early syphilis. A presumptive diagnosis is possible with the use of two types of serologic tests for syphilis: a) nontreponemal (e.g., Venereal Disease Research Laboratory [VDRL] and RPR) and b) treponemal (e.g., fluorescent treponemal antibody absorbed [FTA-ABS] and microhemagglutination assay for antibody to *T. pallidum* [MHA-TP]). The use of only one type of test is insufficient for diagnosis because false-positive nontreponemal test results occasionally occur secondary to various medical conditions. Nontreponemal test antibody titers usually correlate with disease activity, and results should be reported quantitatively. A fourfold change in titer, equivalent to a change of two dilutions (e.g., from 1:16 to 1:4 or from 1:8 to 1:32), usually is considered necessary to demonstrate a clinically significant difference between two nontreponemal test results that were obtained by using the same serologic test. It is expected that the nontreponemal test will eventually become nonreactive after treatment; however, in some patients, nontreponemal antibodies can persist at a low titer for a long period, sometimes for the remainder of their lives. This response is referred to as the serofast reaction. Most patients who have reactive treponemal tests will have reactive tests for the remainder of their lives, regardless of treatment or disease activity. However, 15%–25% of patients treated during the primary stage might revert to being serologically nonreactive after 2–3 years. Treponemal test antibody titers correlate poorly with disease activity and should not be used to assess treatment response.

Sequential serologic tests should be performed by using the same testing method (e.g., VDRL or RPR), preferably by the same laboratory. The VDRL and RPR are equally valid, but quantitative results from the two tests cannot be compared directly because RPR titers often are slightly higher than VDRL titers.

HIV-infected patients can have abnormal serologic test results (i.e., unusually high, unusually low, and fluctuating titers). For such patients with clinical syndromes suggestive of early syphilis, use of other tests (e.g., biopsy and direct microscopy) should be considered. However, for most HIV-infected patients, serologic tests appear to be accurate and reliable for the diagnosis of syphilis and for evaluation of treatment response.

No single test can be used to diagnose all cases of neurosyphilis. The diagnosis of neurosyphilis can be made based on various combinations of reactive serologic test results, abnormalities of cerebrospinal fluid (CSF) cell count or protein, or a reactive VDRL-CSF with or without clinical manifestations. The CSF leukocyte count usually is elevated (>5 WBCs/mm^3) when neurosyphilis is present, and it also is a sensitive measure of the effectiveness of therapy. The VDRL-CSF is the standard serologic test for CSF; when reactive in the absence of substantial contamination of CSF with blood, it is considered diagnostic of neurosyphilis. However, the VDRL-CSF may be nonreactive when neurosyphilis is present. Some experts recommend performing an FTA-ABS test on CSF. The CSF FTA-ABS is less specific (i.e., yields more false-positive results) for neurosyphilis than the VDRL-CSF. However, the test is believed to be highly sensitive, and some experts believe that a negative CSF FTA-ABS test excludes neurosyphilis.

Treatment

Parenteral penicillin G is the preferred drug for treatment of all stages of syphilis. The preparation(s) used (i.e., benzathine, aqueous procaine, or aqueous crystalline), the dosage, and the length of treatment depend on the stage and clinical manifestations of disease.

The efficacy of penicillin for the treatment of syphilis was well established through clinical experience before the value of randomized controlled clinical trials was recognized. Therefore, almost all the recommendations for the treatment of syphilis are based on expert opinion reinforced by case series, clinical trials, and 50 years of clinical experience.

Parenteral penicillin G is the only therapy with documented efficacy for neurosyphilis or for syphilis during pregnancy. Patients who report a penicillin allergy, including pregnant women with syphilis in any stage and patients with neurosyphilis, should be desensitized and treated with penicillin. Skin testing for penicillin allergy may be useful in some settings (see Management of Patients Who Have a History of Penicillin Allergy), because the minor determinants needed for penicillin skin testing are unavailable commercially.

The Jarisch-Herxheimer reaction is an acute febrile reaction—often accompanied by headache, myalgia, and other symptoms—that might occur within the first 24 hours after any therapy for syphilis; patients should be advised of this possible adverse reaction. The Jarisch-Herxheimer reaction often occurs among patients who have early syphilis. Antipyretics may be recommended, but no proven methods prevent this reaction. The Jarisch-Herxheimer reaction may induce early labor or cause fetal distress among pregnant women. This concern should not prevent or delay therapy (see Syphilis During Pregnancy).

Management of Sex Partners

Sexual transmission of *T. pallidum* occurs only when mucocutaneous syphilitic lesions are present; such manifestations are uncommon after the first year of infection. However, persons exposed sexually to a patient who has syphilis in any stage should be evaluated clinically and serologically according to the following recommendations:

- Persons who were exposed within the 90 days preceding the diagnosis of primary, secondary, or early latent syphilis in a sex partner might be infected even if seronegative; therefore, such persons should be treated presumptively.

- Persons who were exposed >90 days before the diagnosis of primary, secondary, or early latent syphilis in a sex partner should be treated presumptively if serologic test results are not available immediately and the opportunity for follow-up is uncertain.

- For purposes of partner notification and presumptive treatment of exposed sex partners, patients with syphilis of unknown duration who have high nontreponemal serologic test titers (i.e., ≥1:32) may be considered as having early syphilis. However, serologic titers should not be used to differentiate early from late latent syphilis for the purpose of determining treatment (see section regarding treatment of latent syphilis).

- Long-term sex partners of patients who have late syphilis should be evaluated clinically and serologically for syphilis and treated on the basis of the findings of the evaluation.

The time periods before treatment used for identifying at-risk sex partners are a) 3 months plus duration of symptoms for primary syphilis, b) 6 months plus duration of symptoms for secondary syphilis, and c) 1 year for early latent syphilis.

Primary and Secondary Syphilis

Treatment
Parenteral penicillin G has been used effectively for four decades to achieve a local cure (i.e., healing of lesions and prevention of sexual transmission) and to prevent late sequelae. However, no adequately conducted comparative trials have been performed to guide the selection of an optimal penicillin regimen (i.e., the dose, duration, and preparation). Substantially fewer data are available concerning nonpenicillin regimens.

Recommended Regimen for Adults
Patients who have primary or secondary syphilis should be treated with the following regimen:

Benzathine penicillin G 2.4 million units IM in a single dose.

NOTE: Recommendations for treating pregnant women and HIV-infected patients for syphilis are discussed in separate sections.

Recommended Regimen for Children
After the newborn period, children in whom syphilis is diagnosed should have a CSF examination to detect asymptomatic neurosyphilis, and birth and maternal medical records should be reviewed to assess whether the child has congenital or acquired syphilis (see Congenital Syphilis). Children with acquired primary or secondary syphilis should be evaluated (including consultation with child-protection services) and treated by using the following pediatric regimen (see Sexual Assault or Abuse of Children).

Benzathine penicillin G 50,000 units/kg IM, up to the adult dose of 2.4 million units in a single dose.

Other Management Considerations
All patients who have syphilis should be tested for HIV infection. In geographic areas in which the prevalence of HIV is high, patients who have primary syphilis should be retested for HIV after 3 months if the first HIV test result was negative. This recommendation will become particularly important if it can be demonstrated that intensive antiviral therapy administered soon after HIV seroconversion is beneficial.

Patients who have syphilis and who also have symptoms or signs suggesting neurologic disease (e.g., meningitis) or ophthalmic disease (e.g., uveitis) should be evaluated fully for neurosyphilis and syphilitic eye disease; this evaluation should include CSF analysis and ocular slit-lamp examination. Such patients should be treated appropriately according to the results of this evaluation.

Invasion of CSF by *T. pallidum* accompanied by CSF abnormalities is common among adults who have primary or secondary syphilis. However, neurosyphilis develops in only a few patients after treatment with the regimens described in this report. Therefore, unless clinical signs or symptoms of neurologic or ophthalmic involvement are present, lumbar puncture is not recommended for routine evaluation of patients who have primary or secondary syphilis.

Follow-Up

Treatment failures can occur with any regimen. However, assessing response to treatment often is difficult, and no definitive criteria for cure or failure have been established. Serologic test titers may decline more slowly for patients who previously had syphilis. Patients should be reexamined clinically and serologically at both 6 months and 12 months; more frequent evaluation may be prudent if follow-up is uncertain.

Patients who have signs or symptoms that persist or recur or who have a sustained fourfold increase in nontreponemal test titer (i.e., in comparison with either the baseline titer or a subsequent result) probably failed treatment or were reinfected. These patients should be re-treated after reevaluation for HIV infection. Unless reinfection with *T. pallidum* is certain, a lumbar puncture also should be performed.

Failure of nontreponemal test titers to decline fourfold within 6 months after therapy for primary or secondary syphilis identifies persons at risk for treatment failure. Such persons should be reevaluated for HIV infection. Optimal management of such patients is unclear. At a minimum, these patients should have additional clinical and serologic follow-up. HIV-infected patients should be evaluated more frequently (i.e., at 3-month intervals instead of 6-month intervals). If additional follow-up cannot be ensured, re-treatment is recommended. Some experts recommend CSF examination in such situations.

When patients are re-treated, most experts recommend re-treatment with three weekly injections of benzathine penicillin G 2.4 million units IM, unless CSF examination indicates that neurosyphilis is present.

Management of Sex Partners

Refer to General Principles, Management of Sex Partners.

Special Considerations

Penicillin Allergy

Nonpregnant penicillin-allergic patients who have primary or secondary syphilis should be treated with one of the following regimens. Close follow-up of such patients is essential.

Recommended Regimens

Doxycycline 100 mg orally twice a day for 2 weeks,
OR
Tetracycline 500 mg orally four times a day for 2 weeks.

There is less clinical experience with doxycycline than with tetracycline, but compliance is likely to be better with doxycycline. Therapy for a patient who cannot tolerate either doxycycline or tetracycline should depend on whether the patient's compliance with the therapy regimen and with follow-up examinations can be ensured.

Pharmacologic and bacteriologic considerations suggest that ceftriaxone should be effective, but data concerning ceftriaxone are limited and clinical experience is insufficient to enable identification of late failures. The optimal dose and duration have not been established for ceftriaxone, but a suggested daily regimen of 1 g may be considered if treponemacidal levels in the blood can be maintained for 8–10 days. Single-dose ceftriaxone therapy is not effective for treating syphilis.

For nonpregnant patients whose compliance with therapy and follow-up can be ensured, an alternative regimen is erythromycin 500 mg orally four times a day for 2 weeks. However, erythromycin is less effective than the other recommended regimens.

Patients whose compliance with therapy or follow-up cannot be ensured should be desensitized and treated with penicillin. Skin testing for penicillin allergy may be useful in some circumstances in which the reagents and expertise to perform the test adequately are available (see Management of Patients Who Have a History of Penicillin Allergy).

Pregnancy

Pregnant patients who are allergic to penicillin should be desensitized, if necessary, and treated with penicillin (see Management of Patients Who Have a History of Penicillin Allergy and Syphilis During Pregnancy).

HIV Infection

Refer to Syphilis in HIV-Infected Persons.

Latent Syphilis

Latent syphilis is defined as those periods after infection with *T. pallidum* when patients are seroreactive, but demonstrate no other evidence of disease. Patients who have latent syphilis and who acquired syphilis within the preceding year are classified as having early latent syphilis. Patients can be demonstrated as having early latent syphilis if, within the year preceding the evaluation, they had a) a documented seroconversion, b) unequivocal symptoms of primary or secondary syphilis, or c) a sex partner who had primary, secondary, or early latent syphilis. Almost all other patients have latent syphilis of unknown duration and should be managed as if they had late latent syphilis. Nontreponemal serologic titers usually are higher during early latent syphilis than late latent syphilis. However, early latent syphilis cannot be reliably distinguished from late latent syphilis solely on the basis of nontreponemal titers. Regardless of the level of the nontreponemal titers, patients in whom the illness does not meet the definition of early syphilis should be treated as if they have late latent infection. All sexually active women with reactive nontreponemal serologic tests should have a pelvic examination before syphilis staging is completed to evaluate for internal mucosal lesions. All patients who have syphilis should be tested for HIV infection.

Treatment

Treatment of latent syphilis is intended to prevent occurrence or progression of late complications. Although clinical experience supports the effectiveness of penicillin in achieving these goals, limited evidence is available for guidance in choosing specific regimens. There is minimal evidence to support the use of non-penicillin regimens.

Recommended Regimens for Adults

The following regimens are recommended for nonallergic patients who have normal CSF examinations (if performed):

Early Latent Syphilis:
Benzathine penicillin G 2.4 million units IM in a single dose.

Late Latent Syphilis or Latent Syphilis of Unknown Duration:
Benzathine penicillin G 7.2 million units total, administered as three doses of 2.4 million units IM each at 1-week intervals.

Recommended Regimens for Children

After the newborn period, children in whom syphilis is diagnosed should have a CSF examination to exclude neurosyphilis, and birth and maternal medical records should be reviewed to assess whether the child has congenital or acquired syphilis (see Congenital Syphilis). Older children with acquired latent syphilis should be evaluated as described for adults and treated using the following pediatric regimens (see Sexual Assault or Abuse of Children). These regimens are for nonallergic children who have acquired syphilis and whose results of the CSF examination were normal.

Early Latent Syphilis:
Benzathine penicillin G 50,000 units/kg IM, up to the adult dose of 2.4 million units in a single dose.

Late Latent Syphilis or Latent Syphilis of Unknown Duration:
Benzathine penicillin G 50,000 units/kg IM, up to the adult dose of 2.4 million units, administered as three doses at 1-week intervals (total 150,000 units/kg up to the adult total dose of 7.2 million units).

Other Management Considerations

All patients who have latent syphilis should be evaluated clinically for evidence of tertiary disease (e.g., aortitis, neurosyphilis, gumma, and iritis). Patients who have syphilis and who demonstrate any of the following criteria should have a prompt CSF examination:

- Neurologic or ophthalmic signs or symptoms;

- Evidence of active tertiary syphilis (e.g., aortitis, gumma, and iritis);

- Treatment failure; and

- HIV infection with late latent syphilis or syphilis of unknown duration.

If dictated by circumstances and patient preferences, a CSF examination may be performed for patients who do not meet these criteria. If a CSF examination is performed and the results indicate abnormalities consistent with neurosyphilis, the patient should be treated for neurosyphilis (see Neurosyphilis).

Follow-Up

Quantitative nontreponemal serologic tests should be repeated at 6, 12, and 24 months. Limited data are available to guide evaluation of the treatment response for patients who have latent syphilis. Patients should be evaluated for neurosyphilis and re-treated appropriately if a) titers increase fourfold, b) an initially high titer ($\geq$1:32) fails to decline at least fourfold (i.e., two dilutions) within 12–24 months, or c) signs or symptoms attributable to syphilis develop in the patient.

Management of Sex Partners

Refer to General Principles, Management of Sex Partners.

Special Considerations

Penicillin Allergy

Nonpregnant patients who have latent syphilis and who are allergic to penicillin should be treated with one of the following regimens.

Recommended Regimens

Doxycycline 100 mg orally twice a day,
OR
Tetracycline 500 mg orally four times a day.

Both drugs should be administered for 2 weeks if the duration of infection is known to have been <1 year; otherwise, they should be administered for 4 weeks.

Pregnancy

Pregnant patients who are allergic to penicillin should be desensitized and treated with penicillin (see Management of Patients Who Have a History of Penicillin Allergy and Syphilis During Pregnancy).

HIV Infection
Refer to Syphilis in HIV-Infected Persons.

Tertiary Syphilis

Tertiary syphilis refers to gumma and cardiovascular syphilis, but not to neuro-syphilis. Nonallergic patients without evidence of neurosyphilis should be treated with the following regimen.

Recommended Regimen
***

Benzathine penicillin G 7.2 million units total, administered as three doses of 2.4 million units IM at 1-week intervals.

***

Other Management Considerations

Patients who have symptomatic late syphilis should have a CSF examination before therapy is initiated. Some experts treat all patients who have cardiovascular syphilis with a neurosyphilis regimen. The complete management of patients who have cardiovascular or gummatous syphilis is beyond the scope of these guide-lines. These patients should be managed in consultation with an expert.

Follow-Up

Information is lacking with regard to follow-up of patients who have late syphi-lis. The clinical response depends partially on the nature of the lesions.

Management of Sex Partners

Refer to General Principles, Management of Sex Partners.

Special Considerations

Penicillin Allergy

Patients allergic to penicillin should be treated according to the recommended regimens for late latent syphilis.

Pregnancy

Pregnant patients who are allergic to penicillin should be desensitized, if neces-sary, and treated with penicillin (see Management of Patients Who Have a History of Penicillin Allergy and Syphilis During Pregnancy).

HIV Infection

Refer to Syphilis in HIV-Infected Persons.

Neurosyphilis

Treatment

Central nervous system disease can occur during any stage of syphilis. A patient who has clinical evidence of neurologic involvement with syphilis (e.g., ophthalmic or auditory symptoms, cranial nerve palsies, and symptoms or signs of meningitis) should have a CSF examination.

Syphilitic uveitis or other ocular manifestations frequently are associated with neurosyphilis; patients with these symptoms should be treated according to the recommendations for neurosyphilis. A CSF examination should be performed for all such patients to identify those with abnormalities who should have follow-up CSF examinations to assess treatment response.

Patients who have neurosyphilis or syphilitic eye disease (e.g., uveitis, neuroretinitis, or optic neuritis) and who are not allergic to penicillin should be treated with the following regimen:

Recommended Regimen

Aqueous crystalline penicillin G 18–24 million units a day, administered as 3–4 million units IV every 4 hours for 10–14 days.

If compliance with therapy can be ensured, patients may be treated with the following alternative regimen:

Alternative Regimen

Procaine penicillin 2.4 million units IM a day, PLUS Probenecid 500 mg orally four times a day, both for 10–14 days.

The durations of the recommended and alternative regimens for neurosyphilis are shorter than that of the regimen used for late syphilis in the absence of neurosyphilis. Therefore, some experts administer benzathine penicillin, 2.4 million units IM, after completion of these neurosyphilis treatment regimens to provide a comparable total duration of therapy.

Other Management Considerations

Other considerations in the management of patients who have neurosyphilis are as follows:

- All patients who have syphilis should be tested for HIV.

- Many experts recommend treating patients who have evidence of auditory disease caused by syphilis in the same manner as for neurosyphilis, regardless of the findings on CSF examination. Although systemic steroids are used frequently as adjunctive therapy for otologic syphilis, such drugs have not been proven beneficial.

Follow-Up

If CSF pleocytosis was present initially, a CSF examination should be repeated every 6 months until the cell count is normal. Follow-up CSF examinations also can be used to evaluate changes in the VDRL-CSF or CSF protein after therapy; however, changes in these two parameters are slower, and persistent abnormalities are of less importance. If the cell count has not decreased after 6 months, or if the CSF is not entirely normal after 2 years, re-treatment should be considered.

Management of Sex Partners

Refer to General Principles, Management of Sex Partners.

Special Considerations

Penicillin Allergy

Data have not been collected systematically for evaluation of therapeutic alternatives to penicillin for treatment of neurosyphilis. Patients who report being allergic to penicillin should either be densensitized to penicillin or be managed in consultation with an expert. In some situations, skin testing to confirm penicillin allergy may be useful (see Management of Patients Who Have a History of Penicillin Allergy).

Pregnancy

Pregnant patients who are allergic to penicillin should be desensitized, if necessary, and treated with penicillin (see Syphilis During Pregnancy).

HIV Infection

Refer to Syphilis in HIV-Infected Persons.

Syphilis in HIV-Infected Persons

Diagnostic Considerations

Unusual serologic responses have been observed among HIV-infected persons who have syphilis. Most reports involved serologic titers that were higher than expected, but false-negative serologic test results or delayed appearance of seroreactivity also have been reported. Nevertheless, both treponemal and nontreponemal serologic tests for syphilis can be interpreted in the usual manner for most patients who are coinfected with *T. pallidum* and HIV.

When clinical findings suggest that syphilis is present, but serologic tests are nonreactive or unclear, alternative tests (e.g., biopsy of a lesion, darkfield examination, or direct fluorescent antibody staining of lesion material) may be useful.

Neurosyphilis should be considered in the differential diagnosis of neurologic disease in HIV-infected persons.

Treatment

In comparison with HIV-negative patients, HIV-infected patients who have early syphilis may be at increased risk for neurologic complications and may have higher rates of treatment failure with currently recommended regimens. The magnitude of these risks, although not defined precisely, is probably minimal. No treatment regimens for syphilis are demonstrably more effective in preventing neurosyphilis in HIV-infected patients than the syphilis regimens recommended for HIV-negative patients. Careful follow-up after therapy is essential.

Primary and Secondary Syphilis in HIV-Infected Persons

Treatment

Treatment with benzathine penicillin G, 2.4 million units IM, as for HIV-negative patients, is recommended. Some experts recommend additional treatments (e.g., three weekly doses of benzathine penicillin G as suggested for late syphilis) or other supplemental antibiotics in addition to benzathine penicillin G 2.4 million units IM.

Other Management Considerations

CSF abnormalities often occur among both asymptomatic HIV-infected patients in the absence of syphilis and HIV-negative patients who have primary or secondary syphilis. Such abnormalities in HIV-infected patients who have primary or secondary syphilis are of unknown prognostic significance. Most HIV-infected patients respond appropriately to the currently recommended penicillin therapy; however, some experts recommend CSF examination before therapy and modification of treatment accordingly.

Follow-Up

It is important that HIV-infected patients be evaluated clinically and serologically for treatment failure at 3, 6, 9, 12, and 24 months after therapy. Although of unproven benefit, some experts recommend a CSF examination after therapy (i.e., at 6 months).

HIV-infected patients who meet the criteria for treatment failure should be managed the same as HIV-negative patients (i.e., a CSF examination and re-treatment). CSF examination and re-treatment also should be strongly considered for patients whose nontreponemal test titer does not decrease fourfold within 6–12 months. Most experts would re-treat patients with 7.2 million units of benzathine penicillin G (administered as three weekly doses of 2.4 million units each) if CSF examinations are normal.

Special Considerations

Penicillin Allergy

Penicillin-allergic patients who have primary or secondary syphilis and HIV infection should be managed according to the recommendations for penicillin-allergic HIV-negative patients.

Latent Syphilis in HIV-Infected Persons

Diagnostic Considerations

HIV-infected patients who have early latent syphilis should be managed and treated according to the recommendations for HIV-negative patients who have primary and secondary syphilis.

HIV-infected patients who have either late latent syphilis or syphilis of unknown duration should have a CSF examination before treatment.

Treatment

A patient with late latent syphilis or syphilis of unknown duration and a normal CSF examination can be treated with 7.2 million units of benzathine penicillin G (as three weekly doses of 2.4 million units each). Patients who have CSF consistent with neurosyphilis should be treated and managed as described for neurosyphilis (see Neurosyphilis).

Follow-Up

Patients should be evaluated clinically and serologically at 6, 12, 18, and 24 months after therapy. If, at any time, clinical symptoms develop or nontreponemal titers rise fourfold, a repeat CSF examination should be performed and treatment administered accordingly. If between 12 and 24 months the nontreponemal titer fails to decline fourfold, the CSF examination should be repeated, and treatment administered accordingly.

Special Considerations

Penicillin Allergy

Penicillin regimens should be used to treat all stages of syphilis in HIV-infected patients. Skin testing to confirm penicillin allergy may be used (see Management of Patients Who Have a History of Penicillin Allergy). Patients may be desensitized, then treated with penicillin.

Syphilis During Pregnancy

All women should be screened serologically for syphilis during the early stages of pregnancy. In populations in which utilization of prenatal care is not optimal, RPR-card test screening and treatment (i.e., if the RPR-card test is reactive) should be performed at the time a pregnancy is diagnosed. For communities and populations in which the prevalence of syphilis is high or for patients at high risk, serologic testing should be performed twice during the third trimester, at 28 weeks of gestation and at delivery. (Some states mandate screening at delivery for all women.) Any woman who delivers a stillborn infant after 20 weeks of gestation should be tested for syphilis. No infant should leave the hospital without the maternal serologic status having been determined at least once during pregnancy.

Diagnostic Considerations

Seropositive pregnant women should be considered infected unless an adequate treatment history is documented clearly in the medical records and sequential serologic antibody titers have declined.

Treatment

Penicillin is effective for preventing maternal transmission to the fetus and for treating fetal-established infection. Evidence is insufficient to determine whether the specific, recommended penicillin regimens are optimal.

Recommended Regimens

Treatment during pregnancy should be the penicillin regimen appropriate for the stage of syphilis.

Other Management Considerations

Some experts recommend additional therapy in some settings. A second dose of benzathine penicillin 2.4 million units IM may be administered 1 week after the initial dose for women who have primary, secondary, or early latent syphilis. Ultrasonographic signs of fetal syphilis (i.e., hepatomegaly and hydrops) indicate a greater risk for fetal treatment failure; such cases should be managed in consultation with obstetric specialists.

Women treated for syphilis during the second half of pregnancy are at risk for premature labor and/or fetal distress if the treatment precipitates the Jarisch-Herxheimer reaction. These women should be advised to seek obstetric attention after treatment if they notice any contractions or decrease in fetal movements. Stillbirth is a rare complication of treatment, but concern for this complication should not delay necessary treatment. All patients who have syphilis should be offered testing for HIV infection.

Follow-Up

Coordinated prenatal care and treatment follow-up are important, and syphilis case management may help facilitate prenatal enrollment. Serologic titers should be repeated in the third trimester and at delivery. Serologic titers may be checked monthly in women at high risk for reinfection or in geographic areas in which the prevalence of syphilis is high. The clinical and antibody response should be appropriate for the stage of disease. Most women will deliver before their serologic response to treatment can be assessed definitively.

Management of Sex Partners

Refer to General Principles, Management of Sex Partners.

Special Considerations

Penicillin Allergy

There are no proven alternatives to penicillin for treatment of syphilis during pregnancy. Pregnant women who have a history of penicillin allergy should be desensitized and treated with penicillin. Skin testing may be helpful (see Management of Patients Who Have a History of Penicillin Allergy).

Tetracycline and doxycycline usually are not used during pregnancy. Erythromycin should not be used, because it does not reliably cure an infected fetus. Data are insufficient to recommend azithromycin or ceftriaxone.

HIV Infection

Refer to Syphilis in HIV-Infected Persons.

CONGENITAL SYPHILIS

Effective prevention and detection of congenital syphilis depends on the identification of syphilis in pregnant women and, therefore, on the routine serologic screening of pregnant women at the time of the first prenatal visit. Serologic testing and a sexual history also should be obtained at 28 weeks of gestation and at delivery in communities and populations in which the risk for congenital syphilis is high. Moreover, as part of the management of pregnant women who have syphilis, information concerning treatment of sex partners should be obtained in order to assess possible maternal reinfection. All pregnant women who have syphilis should be tested for HIV infection.

Routine screening of newborn sera or umbilical cord blood is not recommended. Serologic testing of the mother's serum is preferred to testing infant serum, because the serologic tests performed on infant serum can be nonreactive if the mother's serologic test result is of low titer or if the mother was infected late in pregnancy. No infant should leave the hospital without the maternal serologic status having been documented at least once during pregnancy.

Evaluation and Treatment of Infants During the First Month of Life

Diagnostic Considerations

The diagnosis of congenital syphilis is complicated by the transplacental transfer of maternal nontreponemal and treponemal IgG antibodies to the fetus. This transfer of antibodies makes the interpretation of reactive serologic tests for syphilis in infants difficult. Treatment decisions often must be made based on a) identification of syphilis in the mother; b) adequacy of maternal treatment; c) presence of clinical, laboratory, or radiographic evidence of syphilis in the infant; and d) comparison of the infant's nontreponemal serologic test results with those of the mother.

Who Should Be Evaluated

All infants born to seroreactive mothers should be evaluated with a quantitative nontreponemal serologic test (RPR or VDRL) performed on infant serum (i.e., umbilical cord blood might be contaminated with maternal blood and might yield a false-positive result). A treponemal test (i.e., MHA-TP or FTA-ABS) of a newborn's serum is not necessary.

Evaluation

All infants born to women who have reactive serologic tests for syphilis should be examined thoroughly for evidence of congenital syphilis (e.g., nonimmune hydrops, jaundice, hepatosplenomegaly, rhinitis, skin rash, and/or pseudoparalysis of an extremity). Pathologic examination of the placenta or umbilical cord using specific fluorescent antitreponemal antibody staining is suggested. Darkfield microscopic examination or direct fluorescent antibody staining of suspicious lesions or body fluids (e.g., nasal discharge) also should be performed.

Further evaluation of the infant is dependent on a) whether any abnormalities are present on physical examination, b) maternal treatment history, c) stage of infection at the time of treatment, and d) comparison of maternal (at delivery) and infant nontreponemal titers utilizing the same test and preferably the same laboratory.

Treatment

Infants should be treated for presumed congenital syphilis if they were born to mothers who met any of the following criteria:

- Had untreated syphilis at delivery;*

- Had serologic evidence of relapse or reinfection after treatment (i.e., a fourfold or greater increase in nontreponemal antibody titer);

- Was treated with erythromycin or other nonpenicillin regimen for syphilis during pregnancy;[†]

- Was treated for syphilis ≤1 month before delivery;

- Did not have a well-documented history of treatment for syphilis;

- Was treated for early syphilis during pregnancy with the appropriate penicillin regimen, but nontreponemal antibody titers did not decrease at least fourfold; or

- Was treated appropriately before pregnancy but had insufficient serologic follow-up to ensure an adequate treatment response and lack of current infection (i.e., an appropriate response includes a] at least a fourfold decrease in nontreponemal antibody titers for patients treated for early syphilis and b] stable or declining nontreponemal titers of ≤1:4 for other patients).

Regardless of a maternal history of infection with *T. pallidum* or treatment for syphilis, the evaluation should include the following tests if the infant has either a) an abnormal physical examination that is consistent with congenital syphilis, b) a serum quantitative nontreponemal serologic titer that is fourfold greater than the mother's titer, or c) a positive darkfield or fluorescent antibody test of body fluid(s).

- CSF analysis for VDRL, cell count, and protein;

- Complete blood count (CBC) and differential CBC and platelet count;

- Other tests as clinically indicated (e.g., long-bone radiographs, chest radiograph, liver-function tests, cranial ultrasound, ophthalmologic examination, and auditory brainstem response).

Recommended Regimens

Aqueous crystalline penicillin G 100,000–150,000 units/kg/day, administered as 50,000 units/kg/dose IV every 12 hours during the first 7 days of life, and every 8 hours thereafter for a total of 10 days;

OR

Procaine penicillin G 50,000 units/kg/dose IM a day in a single dose for 10 days.

---

*A woman treated with a regimen other than those recommended in these guidelines for treatment of syphilis should be considered untreated.
†The absence of a fourfold greater titer for an infant does not exclude congenital syphilis.

If >1 day of therapy is missed, the entire course should be restarted. Data are insufficient regarding the use of other antimicrobial agents (e.g., ampicillin). When possible, a full 10-day course of penicillin is preferred. The use of agents other than penicillin requires close serologic follow-up to assess adequacy of therapy.

In all other situations, the maternal history of infection with *T. pallidum* and treatment for syphilis must be considered when evaluating and treating the infant. For infants who have a normal physical examination and a serum quantitative nontreponemal serologic titer the same or less than fourfold the maternal titer, the evaluation depends on the maternal treatment history and stage of infection.

- The infant should receive the following treatment if a) the maternal treatment was not given, was undocumented, was a nonpenicillin regimen, or was administered ≤4 weeks before delivery; b) the adequacy of maternal treatment for early syphilis cannot be evaluated because the nontreponemal serologic titer has not decreased fourfold; or c) relapse or reinfection is suspected because of a fourfold increase in maternal nontreponemal serologic titer.

  a. Aqueous penicillin G or procaine penicillin G for 10 days. Some experts prefer this therapy if the mother has untreated early syphilis at delivery. A complete evaluation is unnecessary if 10 days of parenteral therapy is given. However such evaluation may be useful; a lumbar puncture may document CSF abnormalities that would prompt close follow-up.* Other tests (e.g., CBC and platelet count and bone radiographs) may be performed to further support a diagnosis of congenital syphilis; *or*

  b. Benzathine penicillin G 50,000 units/kg (single dose IM) if the infant's evaluation (i.e., CSF examination, long-bone radiographs, and CBC with platelets) is normal and follow-up is certain. If any part of the infant's evaluation is abnormal or not done, or the CSF analysis is uninterpretable secondary to contamination with blood, then a 10-day course of penicillin (see preceding paragraph) is required.[†]

- Evaluation is unnecessary if the maternal treatment a) was during pregnancy, appropriate for the stage of infection, and >4 weeks before delivery; b) was for early syphilis and the nontreponemal serologic titers decreased fourfold after appropriate therapy; or c) was for late latent infection, the nontreponemal titers remained stable and low, and there is no evidence of maternal reinfection or relapse. A single dose of benzathine penicillin G 50,000 units/kg IM should be administered. (Note: Some experts would not treat the infant but would provide

---

*CSF test results obtained during the neonatal period can be difficult to interpret; normal values differ by gestational age and are higher in preterm infants. Values as high as 25 white blood cells (WBCs)/mm^3 and/or protein of 150 mg/dL might occur among normal neonates; some experts, however, recommend that lower values (i.e., 5 WBCs/mm^3 and protein of 40 mg/dL) be considered the upper limits of normal. Other causes of elevated values also should be considered when an infant is being evaluated for congenital syphilis.

[†]If the infant's nontreponemal test is nonreactive and the likelihood of the infant being infected is low, some experts recommend no evaluation but treatment of the infant with a single IM dose of benzathine penicillin G 50,000 units/kg for possible incubating syphilis, after which the infant should have close serologic follow-up.

close serologic follow-up.) Furthermore, in these situations, if the infant's non-treponemal test is nonreactive, no treatment is necessary.

- Evaluation and treatment are unnecessary if the maternal treatment was before pregnancy, after which the mother was evaluated multiple times, and the nontreponemal serologic titer remained low and stable before and during pregnancy and at delivery (VDRL ≤1:2; RPR ≤1:4). Some experts would treat with benzathine penicillin G 50,000 units/kg as a single IM injection, particularly if follow-up is uncertain.

Evaluation and Treatment of Older Infants and Children Who Have Congenital Syphilis

Children who are identified as having reactive serologic tests for syphilis after the neonatal period (i.e., at >1 month of age) should have maternal serology and records reviewed to assess whether the child has congenital or acquired syphilis (for acquired syphilis, see Primary and Secondary Syphilis and Latent Syphilis). If the child possibly has congenital syphilis, the child should be evaluated fully (i.e., a CSF examination for cell count, protein, and VDRL [abnormal CSF evaluation includes a reactive VDRL test, >5 WBCs/mm^3, and/or protein >40 mg/dL]; an eye examination; and other tests such as long-bone radiographs, CBC, platelet count, and auditory brainstem response as indicated clinically). Any child who possibly has congenital syphilis or who has neurologic involvement should be treated with aqueous crystalline penicillin G, 200,000–300,000 units/kg/day IV (administered as 50,000 units/kg every 4–6 hours) for 10 days.

Follow-Up

All seroreactive infants (or an infant whose mother was seroreactive at delivery) should receive careful follow-up examinations and serologic testing (i.e., a nontreponemal test) every 2–3 months until the test becomes nonreactive or the titer has decreased fourfold. Nontreponemal antibody titers should decline by 3 months of age and should be nonreactive by 6 months of age if the infant was not infected (i.e., if the reactive test result was caused by passive transfer of maternal IgG antibody) or was infected but adequately treated. The serologic response after therapy may be slower for infants treated after the neonatal period. If these titers are stable or increasing after 6–12 months of age, the child should be evaluated, including a CSF examination, and treated with a 10-day course of parenteral penicillin G.

Treponemal tests should not be used to evaluate treatment response because the results for an infected child can remain positive despite effective therapy. Passively transferred maternal treponemal antibodies could be present in an infant until age 15 months. A reactive treponemal test after age 18 months is diagnostic of congenital syphilis. If the nontreponemal test is nonreactive at this time, no further evaluation or treatment is necessary. If the nontreponemal test is reactive at age 18 months, the infant should be fully (re)evaluated and treated for congenital syphilis.

Infants whose initial CSF evaluation is abnormal should undergo a repeat lumbar puncture approximately every 6 months until the results are normal. A reactive CSF VDRL test or abnormal CSF indices that cannot be attributed to other ongoing illness requires re-treatment for possible neurosyphilis.

Follow-up of children treated for congenital syphilis after the newborn period should be the same as that prescribed for congenital syphilis among neonates.

Special Considerations

Penicillin Allergy

Infants and children who require treatment for syphilis but who have a history of penicillin allergy or develop an allergic reaction presumed secondary to penicillin should be desensitized, if necessary, and treated with penicillin. Skin testing may be helpful in some patients and settings (see Management of Patients Who Have a History of Penicillin Allergy). Data are insufficient regarding the use of other antimicrobial agents (e.g., ceftriaxone); if a nonpenicillin agent is used, close serologic and CSF follow-up is indicated.

HIV Infection

Data are insufficient regarding whether infants who have congenital syphilis and whose mothers are coinfected with HIV require different evaluation, therapy, or follow-up for syphilis than is recommended for all infants.

MANAGEMENT OF PATIENTS WHO HAVE A HISTORY OF PENICILLIN ALLERGY

No proven alternatives to penicillin are available for treating neurosyphilis, congenital syphilis, or syphilis in pregnant women. Penicillin also is recommended for use, whenever possible, in HIV-infected patients. Of the adult U.S. population, 3%–10% have experienced urticaria, angioedema, or anaphylaxis (i.e., upper airway obstruction, bronchospasm, or hypotension) after penicillin therapy. Re-administration of penicillin to these patients can cause severe, immediate reactions. Because anaphylactic reactions to penicillin can be fatal, every effort should be made to avoid administering penicillin to penicillin-allergic patients, unless the anaphylactic sensitivity has been removed by acute desensitization.

An estimated 10% of persons who report a history of severe allergic reactions to penicillin are still allergic. With the passage of time after an allergic reaction to penicillin, most persons who have had a severe reaction stop expressing penicillin-specific IgE. These persons can be treated safely with penicillin. The results of many investigations indicate that skin testing with the major and minor determinants can reliably identify persons at high risk for penicillin reactions. Although these reagents are easily generated and have been available in academic centers for >30 years, only benzylpenicilloyl poly-L-lysine (Pre-Pen, the major determinant) and penicillin G are available commercially. Experts estimate that testing with only the major determinant and penicillin G identifies 90%–97% of the currently allergic patients. However, because skin testing without the minor determinants would still miss 3%–10% of allergic patients, and serious or fatal reactions can occur among these minor-determinant–positive patients, experts suggest caution when the full battery of skin-test reagents is not available (Table 1).

Recommendations

If the full battery of skin-test reagents is available, including the major and minor determinants (see Penicillin Allergy Skin Testing), patients who report a history of penicillin reaction and are skin-test negative can receive conventional penicillin therapy. Skin-test–positive patients should be desensitized.

If the full battery of skin-test reagents, including the minor determinants, is not available, the patient should be skin tested using benzylpenicilloyl poly-L-lysine (i.e., the major determinant, Pre-Pen) and penicillin G. Patients who have positive test results should be desensitized. Some experts believe that persons who have negative test results should be regarded as probably allergic and should be desensitized. Others suggest that those with negative skin-test results can be test-dosed gradually with oral penicillin in a monitored setting in which treatment for anaphylactic reaction is possible.

TABLE 1. Oral desensitization protocol for patients with a positive skin test*

Penicillin V suspension dose[†]	Amount[§] (units/mL)	mL	Units	Cumulative dose (units)
1	1,000	0.1	100	100
2	1,000	0.2	200	300
3	1,000	0.4	400	700
4	1,000	0.8	800	1,500
5	1,000	1.6	1,600	3,100
6	1,000	3.2	3,200	6,300
7	1,000	6.4	6,400	12,700
8	10,000	1.2	12,000	24,700
9	10,000	2.4	24,000	48,700
10	10,000	4.8	48,000	96,700
11	80,000	1.0	80,000	176,700
12	80,000	2.0	160,000	336,700
13	80,000	4.0	320,000	656,700
14	80,000	8.0	640,000	1,296,700

Observation period: 30 minutes before parenteral administration of penicillin.

*Reprinted with permission from the *New England Journal of Medicine* (*24*).
[†]Interval between doses, 15 minutes; elapsed time, 3 hours and 45 minutes; cumulative dose, 1.3 million units.
[§]The specific amount of drug was diluted in approximately 30 mL of water and then administered orally.

Penicillin Allergy Skin Testing

Patients at high risk for anaphylaxis (i.e., those who have a history of penicillin-related anaphylaxis, asthma, or other diseases that would make anaphylaxis more dangerous or who are being treated with beta-adrenergic blocking agents) should be tested with 100-fold dilutions of the full-strength skin-test reagents before being tested with full-strength reagents. In these situations, patients should be tested in a monitored setting in which treatment for an anaphylactic reaction is available. If possible, the patient should not have taken antihistamines recently (e.g., chlorpheniramine maleate or terfenadine during the preceding 24 hours, diphenhydramine HCl or hydroxyzine during the preceding 4 days, or astemizole during the preceding 3 weeks).

Reagents (Adapted from Beall [25]) *

Major Determinant

- Benzylpenicilloyl poly-L-lysine (Pre-Pen [Taylor Pharmacal Company, Decatur, Illinois]) (6×10^{-5}M).

Minor Determinant Precursors[†]

- Benzylpenicillin G (10^{-2}M, 3.3 mg/mL, 6000 units/mL),

- Benzylpenicilloate (10^{-2}M, 3.3 mg/mL),

- Benzylpenilloate (or penicilloyl propylamine) (10^{-2}M, 3.3 mg/mL).

Positive Control

- Commercial histamine for epicutaneous skin testing (1 mg/mL).

Negative Control

- Diluent used to dissolve other reagents, usually phenol saline.

Procedures

Dilute the antigens a) 100-fold for preliminary testing if the patient has had a life-threatening reaction to penicillin or b) 10-fold if the patient has had another type of immediate, generalized reaction to penicillin within the preceding year.

Epicutaneous (prick) tests. Duplicate drops of skin-test reagent are placed on the volar surface of the forearm. The underlying epidermis is pierced with a 26-gauge needle without drawing blood.

An epicutaneous test is positive if the average wheal diameter after 15 minutes is 4 mm larger than that of negative controls; otherwise, the test is negative. The histamine controls should be positive to ensure that results are not falsely negative because of the effect of antihistaminic drugs.

---

*Reprinted with permission from G.N. Beall in *Annals of Internal Medicine* (*25*).
[†]Aged penicillin is not an adequate source of minor determinants. Penicillin G should be freshly prepared or should come from a fresh-frozen source.

Intradermal tests. If epicutaneous tests are negative, duplicate 0.02 mL intradermal injections of negative control and antigen solutions are made into the volar surface of the forearm using a 26- or 27-gauge needle on a syringe. The crossed diameters of the wheals induced by the injections should be recorded.

An intradermal test is positive if the average wheal diameter 15 minutes after injection is ≥2 mm larger than the initial wheal size and also is ≥2 mm larger than the negative controls. Otherwise, the tests are negative.

Desensitization

Patients who have a positive skin test to one of the penicillin determinants can be desensitized. This is a straightforward, relatively safe procedure that can be done orally or IV. Although the two approaches have not been compared, oral desensitization is regarded as safer to use and easier to perform. Patients should be desensitized in a hospital setting because serious IgE-mediated allergic reactions, although unlikely, can occur. Desensitization usually can be completed in approximately 4 hours, after which the first dose of penicillin is given (Table 1). STD programs should have a referral center where patients who have positive skin test results can be desensitized. After desensitization, patients must be maintained on penicillin continuously for the duration of the course of therapy.

DISEASES CHARACTERIZED BY URETHRITIS AND CERVICITIS

Management of Male Patients Who Have Urethritis

Urethritis, or inflammation of the urethra, is caused by an infection characterized by the discharge of mucopurulent or purulent material and by burning during urination. Asymptomatic infections are common. The only bacterial pathogens of proven clinical importance in men who have urethritis are *N. gonorrhoeae* and *C. trachomatis*. Testing to determine the specific disease is recommended because both of these infections are reportable to state health departments, and a specific diagnosis may improve compliance and partner notification. If diagnostic tools (e.g., a Gram stain and microscope) are unavailable, patients should be treated for both infections. The extra expense of treating a person who has nongonococcal urethritis (NGU) for both infections also should encourage the health-care provider to make a specific diagnosis. New nucleic acid amplification tests enable detection of *N. gonorrhoeae* and *C. trachomatis* on first-void urine; in some settings, these tests are more sensitive than traditional culture techniques.

Etiology

NGU is diagnosed if Gram-negative intracellular organisms cannot be identified on Gram stains. *C. trachomatis* is the most frequent cause (i.e., in 23%–55% of cases); however, the prevalence differs by age group, with lower prevalence among older men. The proportion of NGU cases caused by chlamydia has been declining gradually. Complications of NGU among men infected with *C. trachomatis* include epididymitis and Reiter's syndrome. Documentation of chlamydia infection is important because partner referral for evaluation and treatment would be indicated.

The etiology of most cases of nonchlamydial NGU is unknown. *Ureaplasma urealyticum* and possibly *Mycoplasma genitalium* are implicated in as many as one third of cases. Specific diagnostic tests for these organisms are not indicated.

Trichomonas vaginalis and HSV sometimes cause NGU. Diagnostic and treatment procedures for these organisms are reserved for situations in which NGU is nonresponsive to therapy.

Confirmed Urethritis

Clinicians should document that urethritis is present. Urethritis can be documented by the presence of any of the following signs:

a. Mucopurulent or purulent discharge.
b. Gram stain of urethral secretions demonstrating ≥5 WBCs per oil immersion field. The Gram stain is the preferred rapid diagnostic test for evaluating urethritis. It is highly sensitive and specific for documenting both urethritis and the presence or absence of gonococcal infection. Gonococcal infection is established by documenting the presence of WBCs containing intracellular Gram-negative diplococci.
c. Positive leukocyte esterase test on first-void urine, or microscopic examination of first-void urine demonstrating ≥10 WBCs per high power field.

If none of these criteria is present, then treatment should be deferred, and the patient should be tested for *N. gonorrhoeae* and *C. trachomatis* and followed closely in the event of a positive test result. If the results demonstrate infection with either *N. gonorrhoeae* or *C. trachomatis*, the appropriate treatment should be given and sex partners referred for evaluation and treatment.

Empiric treatment of symptoms without documentation of urethritis is recommended only for patients at high risk for infection who are unlikely to return for a follow-up evaluation (e.g., adolescents who have multiple partners). Such patients should be treated for gonorrhea and chlamydia. Partners of patients treated empirically should be referred for evaluation and treatment.

Management of Patients Who Have Nongonococcal Urethritis

Diagnosis

All patients who have urethritis should be evaluated for the presence of gonococcal and chlamydial infection. Testing for chlamydia is strongly recommended because of the increased utility and availability of highly sensitive and specific testing methods and because a specific diagnosis might improve compliance and partner notification.

Treatment

Treatment should be initiated as soon as possible after diagnosis. Single-dose regimens have the important advantage of improved compliance and of directly observed therapy. If multiple-dose regimens are used, the medication should be provided in the clinic or health-care provider's office. Treatment with the recommended regimen can result in alleviation of symptoms and microbiologic cure of infection.

Recommended Regimens

Azithromycin 1 g orally in a single dose,

OR

Doxycycline 100 mg orally twice a day for 7 days.

Alternative Regimens

Erythromycin base 500 mg orally four times a day for 7 days

OR

Erythromycin ethylsuccinate 800 mg orally four times a day for 7 days,

OR

Ofloxacin 300 mg twice a day for 7 days.

If only erythromycin can be used and a patient cannot tolerate high-dose erythromycin schedules, one of the following regimens can be used:

Erythromycin base 250 mg orally four times a day for 14 days,

OR

Erythromycin ethylsuccinate 400 mg orally four times a day for 14 days.

Follow-Up for Patients Who Have Urethritis

Patients should be instructed to return for evaluation if symptoms persist or recur after completion of therapy. Symptoms alone, without documentation of signs or laboratory evidence of urethral inflammation, are not a sufficient basis for retreatment. Patients should be instructed to abstain from sexual intercourse until therapy is completed.

Partner Referral

Patients should refer for evaluation and treatment all sex partners within the preceding 60 days. A specific diagnosis may facilitate partner referral; therefore, testing for gonorrhea and chlamydia is encouraged.

Recurrent and Persistent Urethritis

Objective signs of urethritis should be present before initiation of antimicrobial therapy. Effective regimens have not been identified for treating patients who have persistent symptoms or frequent recurrences after treatment. Patients who have persistent or recurrent urethritis should be re-treated with the initial regimen if they did not comply with the treatment regimen or if they were reexposed to an untreated sex partner. Otherwise, a wet mount examination and culture of an intraurethral swab specimen for *T. vaginalis* should be performed. Urologic examinations usually do not reveal a specific etiology. If the patient was compliant with the initial regimen and reexposure can be excluded, the following regimen is recommended:

Recommended Treatment for Recurrent/Persistent Urethritis

Metronidazole 2 g orally in a single dose,
PLUS
Erythromycin base 500 mg orally four times a day for 7 days,
OR
Erythromycin ethylsuccinate 800 mg orally four times a day for 7 days.

Special Considerations

HIV Infection

Gonococcal urethritis, chlamydial urethritis, and nongoncoccal, nonchlamydial urethritis may facilitate HIV transmission. Patients who have NGU and also are infected with HIV should receive the same treatment regimen as those who are HIV-negative.

Management of Patients Who Have Mucopurulent Cervicitis (MPC)

MPC is characterized by a purulent or mucopurulent endocervical exudate visible in the endocervical canal or in an endocervical swab specimen. Some experts also make the diagnosis on the basis of easily induced cervical bleeding. Although some experts consider an increased number of polymorphonuclear leukocytes on endocervical Gram stain as being useful in the diagnosis of MPC, this criterion has not been standardized, has a low positive-predictive value (PPV), and is not available in some settings. MPC often is asymptomatic, but some women have an abnormal vaginal discharge and vaginal bleeding (e.g., after sexual intercourse). MPC can be caused by *C. trachomatis* or *N. gonorrhoeae*; however, in most cases neither organism can be isolated. MPC can persist despite repeated courses of antimicrobial therapy. Because relapse or reinfection with *C. trachomatis* or *N. gonorrhoeae* usually does not apply to persistent cases of MPC, other nonmicrobiologic determinants (e.g., inflammation in an ectropion) could be involved.

Patients who have MPC should be tested for *C. trachomatis* and for *N. gonorrhoeae* by using the most sensitive and specific test for the population served. However, MPC is not a sensitive predictor of infection with these organisms, because most women who have *C. trachomatis* or *N. gonorrhoeae* do not have MPC.

Treatment

The results of sensitive tests for *C. trachomatis* or *N. gonorrhoeae* (e.g., culture or nucleic acid amplification tests) should determine the need for treatment, unless the likelihood of infection with either organism is high or the patient is unlikely to return for treatment. Empiric treatment should be considered for a patient who has a suspected case of gonorrhea and/or chlamydia if a) the prevalence of these diseases differs substantially (i.e., >15%) between clinics in the geographic area and b) the patient might be difficult to locate for treatment. After the possibilities of relapse and reinfection have been excluded, management of persistent MPC is unclear. For such cases, additional antimicrobial therapy may be of little benefit.

Follow-Up

Follow-up should be as recommended for the infections for which the woman is being treated. If symptoms persist, women should be instructed to return for re-evaluation and to abstain from sexual intercourse even if they have completed the prescribed therapy.

Management of Sex Partners

Management of sex partners of women treated for MPC should be appropriate for the identified or suspected STD. Partners should be notified, examined, and treated for the STD identified or suspected in the index patient.

Patients should be instructed to abstain from sexual intercourse until they and their sex partners are cured. Because a microbiologic test of cure usually is not recommended, patients should abstain from sexual intercourse until therapy is completed (i.e., 7 days after a single-dose regimen or after completion of a 7-day regimen).

Special Considerations

HIV Infection

Patients who have MPC and also are infected with HIV should receive the same treatment regimen as those who are HIV-negative.

Chlamydial Infection

In the United States, chlamydial genital infection occurs frequently among sexually active adolescents and young adults. Asymptomatic infection is common among both men and women. Screening sexually active adolescents for chlamydial infection should be routine during annual examinations, even if symptoms are not present. Screening women aged 20–24 years also is suggested, particularly for those who have new or multiple sex partners and who do not consistently use barrier contraceptives.

Chlamydial Infection in Adolescents and Adults

Several important sequelae can result from *C. trachomatis* infection in women; the most serious of these include PID, ectopic pregnancy, and infertility. Some women who have apparently uncomplicated cervical infection already have subclinical upper reproductive tract infection. A recent investigation of patients in a health maintenance organization demonstrated that screening and treatment of cervical infection can reduce the likelihood of PID.

Treatment

Treatment of infected patients prevents transmission to sex partners; and, for infected pregnant women, treatment might prevent transmission of *C. trachomatis* to infants during birth. Treatment of sex partners helps to prevent reinfection of the index patient and infection of other partners.

Coinfection with *C. trachomatis* often occurs among patients who have gonococcal infection; therefore, presumptive treatment of such patients for chlamydia is appropriate (see Gonococcal Infection, Dual Therapy for Gonococcal and Chlamydial Infections). The following recommended treatment regimens and the alternative regimens cure infection and usually relieve symptoms.

Recommended Regimens

Azithromycin 1 g orally in a single dose,
OR
Doxycycline 100 mg orally twice a day for 7 days.

Alternative Regimens

Erythromycin base 500 mg orally four times a day for 7 days,
OR
Erythromycin ethylsuccinate 800 mg orally four times a day for 7 days,
OR
Ofloxacin 300 mg orally twice a day for 7 days.

The results of clinical trials indicate that azithromycin and doxycycline are equally efficacious. These investigations were conducted primarily in populations in which follow-up was encouraged and adherence to a 7-day regimen was good. Azithromycin should always be available to health-care providers to treat at least those patients for whom compliance is in question.

In populations with erratic health-care–seeking behavior, poor compliance with treatment, or minimal follow-up, azithromycin may be more cost-effective because it provides single-dose, directly observed therapy. Doxycycline costs less than azithromycin, and it has been used extensively for a longer period. Erythromycin is less efficacious than either azithromycin and doxycycline, and gastrointestinal side effects frequently discourage patients from complying with this regimen. Ofloxacin is similar in efficacy to doxycycline and azithromycin, but it is more expensive to use and offers no advantage with regard to the dosage regimen. Other quinolones either are not reliably effective against chlamydial infection or have not been adequately evaluated.

To maximize compliance with recommended therapies, medications for chlamydial infections should be dispensed on site, and the first dose should be directly observed. To minimize further transmission of infection, patients treated for chlamydia should be instructed to abstain from sexual intercourse for 7 days after single-dose therapy or until completion of a 7-day regimen. Patients also should be instructed to abstain from sexual intercourse until all of their sex partners are cured to minimize the risk for reinfection.

Follow-Up

Patients do not need to be retested for chlamydia after completing treatment with doxycycline or azithromycin unless symptoms persist or reinfection is suspected, because these therapies are highly efficacious. A test of cure may be considered 3 weeks after completion of treatment with erythromycin. The validity of chlamydial culture testing at <3 weeks after completion of therapy to identify patients who did not respond to therapy has not been established. False-negative results can occur because of small numbers of chlamydial organisms. In addition, nonculture tests conducted at <3 weeks after completion of therapy for patients who were treated successfully could be false-positive because of continued excretion of dead organisms.

Some studies have demonstrated high rates of infection among women retested several months after treatment, presumably because of reinfection. In some populations (e.g., adolescents), rescreening women several months after treatment might be effective for detecting further morbidity.

Management of Sex Partners

Patients should be instructed to refer their sex partners for evaluation, testing, and treatment. Because exposure intervals have received limited evaluation, the following recommendations are somewhat arbitrary. Sex partners should be evaluated, tested, and treated if they had sexual contact with the patient during the 60 days preceding onset of symptoms in the patient or diagnosis of chlamydia. Health-care providers should treat the most recent sex partner even if the time of the last sexual contact was >60 days before onset or diagnosis.

Patients should be instructed to abstain from sexual intercourse until they and their sex partners have completed treatment. Because a microbiologic test of cure usually is not recommended, abstinence should be continued until therapy is completed (i.e., 7 days after a single-dose regimen or after completion of a 7-day regimen). Timely treatment of sex partners is essential for decreasing the risk for reinfecting the index patient.

Special Considerations
Pregnancy

Doxycycline and ofloxacin are contraindicated for pregnant women. The safety and efficacy of azithromycin use in pregnant and lactating women have not been established. Repeat testing, preferably by culture, 3 weeks after completion of therapy with the following regimens is recommended, because a) none of these regimens are highly efficacious and b) the frequent side effects of erythromycin might discourage patient compliance with this regimen.

Recommended Regimens for Pregnant Women

Erythromycin base 500 mg orally four times a day for 7 days,

OR

Amoxicillin 500 mg orally three times a day for 7 days.

Alternative Regimens for Pregnant Women

Erythromycin base 250 mg orally four times a day for 14 days,

OR

Erythromycin ethylsuccinate 800 mg orally four times a day for 7 days,

OR

Erythromycin ethylsuccinate 400 mg orally four times a day for 14 days,

OR

Azithromycin 1 g orally in a single dose.

Note: Erythromycin estolate is contraindicated during pregnancy because of drug-related hepatotoxicity. Preliminary data indicate that azithromycin may be safe and effective. However, data are insufficient to recommend the routine use of azithromycin in pregnant women.

HIV Infection

Patients who have chlamydial infection and also are infected with HIV should receive the same treatment regimen as those who are HIV-negative.

Chlamydial Infection in Infants

Prenatal screening of pregnant women can prevent chlamydial infection among neonates. Pregnant women who are <25 years of age or who have new or multiple sex partners particularly should be targeted for screening. Periodic prevalence surveys of chlamydial infection can be conducted to confirm the validity of using these recommendations in specific clinical settings.

C. trachomatis infection of neonates results from perinatal exposure to the mother's infected cervix. The prevalence of *C. trachomatis* infection among pregnant women usually is >5%, regardless of race/ethnicity or socioeconomic status. Neonatal ocular prophylaxis with silver nitrate solution or antibiotic ointments does not prevent perinatal transmission of *C. trachomatis* from mother to infant.

However, ocular prophylaxis with those agents does prevent gonoccocal ophthalmia and should be continued for that reason (see Prevention of Ophthalmia Neonatorum).

Initial *C. trachomatis* perinatal infection involves mucous membranes of the eye, oropharynx, urogenital tract, and rectum. *C. trachomatis* infection in neonates is most often recognized by conjunctivitis that develops 5–12 days after birth. Chlamydia is the most frequent identifiable infectious cause of ophthalmia neonatorum. *C. trachomatis* also is a common cause of subacute, afebrile pneumonia with onset from 1 to 3 months of age. Asymptomatic infections also can occur in the oropharynx, genital tract, and rectum of neonates.

Ophthalmia Neonatorum Caused by *C. trachomatis*

A chlamydial etiology should be considered for all infants aged ≤30 days who have conjunctivitis.

Diagnostic Considerations

Sensitive and specific methods used to diagnose chlamydial ophthalmia in the neonate include both tissue culture and nonculture tests (e.g., direct fluorescent antibody tests and immunoassays). Giemsa-stained smears are specific for *C. trachomatis*, but such tests are not sensitive. Specimens must contain conjunctival cells, not exudate alone. Specimens for culture isolation and nonculture tests should be obtained from the everted eyelid using a dacron-tipped swab or the swab specified by the manufacturer's test kit. A specific diagnosis of *C. trachomatis* infection confirms the need for treatment not only for the neonate, but also for the mother and her sex partner(s). Ocular exudate from infants being evaluated for chlamydial conjunctivitis also should be tested for *N. gonorrhoeae*.

Recommended Regimen

Erythromycin 50 mg/kg/day orally divided into four doses daily for 10–14 days.

Topical antibiotic therapy alone is inadequate for treatment of chlamydial infection and is unnecessary when systemic treatment is administered.

Follow-Up

The efficacy of erythromycin treatment is approximately 80%; a second course of therapy may be required. Follow-up of infants to determine resolution is recommended. The possibility of concomitant chlamydial pneumonia should be considered.

Management of Mothers and Their Sex Partners

The mothers of infants who have chlamydial infection and the sex partners of these women should be evaluated and treated (see Chlamydial Infection in Adolescents and Adults).

Infant Pneumonia Caused by *C. trachomatis*

Characteristic signs of chlamydial pneumonia in infants include a) a repetitive staccato cough with tachypnea and b) hyperinflation and bilateral diffuse infiltrates on a chest radiograph. Wheezing is rare, and infants are typically afebrile. Peripheral eosinophilia sometimes occurs in infants who have chlamydial pneumonia. Because clinical presentations differ, initial treatment and diagnostic tests should encompass *C. trachomatis* for all infants aged 1–3 months who possibly have pneumonia.

Diagnostic Considerations

Specimens for chlamydial testing should be collected from the nasopharynx. Tissue culture is the definitive standard for chlamydial pneumonia; nonculture tests can be used with the knowledge that nonculture tests of nasopharyngeal specimens produce lower sensitivity and specificity than nonculture tests of ocular specimens. Tracheal aspirates and lung biopsy specimens, if collected, should be tested for *C. trachomatis*.

The microimmunofluorescence test for *C. trachomatis* antibody is useful but not widely available. An acute IgM antibody titer ≥1:32 is strongly suggestive of *C. trachomatis* pneumonia.

Because of the delay in obtaining test results for chlamydia, the decision to include an agent in the antibiotic regimen that is active against *C. trachomatis* must frequently be based on the clinical and radiologic findings. The results of tests for chlamydial infection assist in the management of an infant's illness and determine the need for treating the mother and her sex partner(s).

Recommended Regimen

Erythromycin base 50 mg/kg/day orally divided into four doses daily for 10–14 days.

Follow-Up

The effectiveness of erythromycin treatment is approximately 80%; a second course of therapy may be required. Follow-up of infants is recommended to determine whether the pneumonia has resolved. Some infants with chlamydial pneumonia have had abnormal pulmonary function tests later in childhood.

Management of Mothers and Their Sex Partners

Mothers of infants who have chlamydial infection and the sex partners of these women should be evaluated and treated according to the recommended treatment of adults for chlamydial infections (see Chlamydial Infection in Adolescents and Adults).

Infants Born to Mothers Who Have Chlamydial Infection

Infants born to mothers who have untreated chlamydia are at high risk for infection; however, prophylatic antibiotic treatment is not indicated, and the efficacy of such treatment is unknown. Infants should be monitored to ensure appropriate treatment if infection develops.

Chlamydial Infection in Children

Sexual abuse must be considered a cause of chlamydial infection in preadolescent children, although perinatally transmitted *C. trachomatis* infection of the nasopharynx, urogenital tract, and rectum may persist for >1 year (see Sexual Assault or Abuse of Children). Because of the potential for a criminal investigation and legal proceedings for sexual abuse, a diagnosis of *C. trachomatis* in a preadolescent child requires the high specificity provided by isolation in cell culture. The cultures should be confirmed by microscopic identification of the characteristic intracytoplasmic inclusions, preferably by fluorescein-conjugated monoclonal antibodies specific for *C. trachomatis*.

Diagnostic Considerations

Nonculture tests for chlamydia should not be used because of the possibility of false-positive test results. With respiratory tract specimens, false-positive results can occur because of cross-reaction of test reagents with *Chlamydia pneumoniae*; with genital and anal specimens, false-positive results occur because of cross-reaction with fecal flora.

Recommended Regimens

Children who weigh <45 kg:
>   **Erythromycin base** 50 mg/kg/day orally divided into four doses daily for 10–14 days.

>   **NOTE:** The effectiveness of treatment with erythromycin is approximately 80%; a second course of therapy may be required.

Children who weigh ≥45 kg but are <8 years of age:
>   **Azithromycin** 1 g orally in a single dose.

Children ≥8 years of age:
>   **Azithromycin** 1 g orally in a single dose,
>   **OR**
>   **Doxycycline** 100 mg orally twice a day for 7 days.

Other Management Considerations

See Sexual Assault or Abuse of Children.

Follow-Up

Follow-up cultures are necessary to ensure that treatment has been effective.

Gonococcal Infection

Gonococcal Infection in Adolescents and Adults

In the United States, an estimated 600,000 new infections with *N. gonorrhoeae* occur each year. Most infections among men produce symptoms that cause them to seek curative treatment soon enough to prevent serious sequelae—but this may not be soon enough to prevent transmission to others. Many infections among women do not produce recognizable symptoms until complications (e.g., pelvic in-flammatory disease [PID]) have occurred. Both symptomatic and asymptomatic cases of PID can result in tubal scarring that leads to infertility or ectopic pregnancy. Because gonococcal infections among women often are asymptomatic, an important component of gonorrhea control in the United States continues to be the screening of women at high risk for STDs.

Dual Therapy for Gonococcal and Chlamydial Infections

Patients infected with *N. gonorrhoeae* often are coinfected with *C. trachomatis*; this finding led to the recommendation that patients treated for gonococcal infection also be treated routinely with a regimen effective against uncomplicated genital *C. trachomatis* infection. Routine dual therapy without testing for chlamydia can be cost-effective for populations in which chlamydial infection accompanies 20%–40% of gonococcal infections, because the cost of therapy for chlamydia (e.g., $0.50–$1.50 for doxycycline) is less than the cost of testing. Some experts believe that the routine use of dual therapy has resulted in substantial decreases in the prevalence of chlamydial infection. Because most gonococci in the United States are susceptible to doxycycline and azithromycin, routine cotreatment might hinder the development of antimicrobial-resistant *N. gonorrhoeae*.

Since the introduction of dual therapy, the prevalence of chlamydial infection has decreased in some populations, and simultaneous testing for chlamydial infection has become quicker, more sensitive, and more widely available. In geographic areas in which the rates of coinfection are low, some clinicians might prefer to test for chlamydia rather than treat presumptively. However, presumptive treatment is indicated for patients who may not return for test results.

Quinolone-Resistant *N. gonorrhoeae* (QRNG)

Cases of gonorrhea caused by *N. gonorrhoeae* resistant to fluoroquinolones have been reported sporadically from many parts of the world, including North America, and are becoming widespread in parts of Asia. As of February 1997, however, QRNG occurred rarely in the United States: <0.05% of 4,639 isolates collected by CDC's Gonococcal Isolate Surveillance Project (GISP) during 1996 had minimum inhibitory concentrations (MICs) ≥1.0 µg/mL to ciprofloxacin. The GISP sample is collected from 26 cities and includes approximately 1.3% of all reported gonococcal infections among men in the United States. As long as QRNG strains comprise <1% of all *N. gonorrhoeae* strains isolated at each of the 26 cities, the fluoroquinolone regimens can be used with confidence. However, importation of QRNG will probably continue, and the prevalence of QRNG in the United States could increase to the point that fluoroquinolones no longer reliably eradicate gonococcal infections.

Uncomplicated Gonococcal Infections of the Cervix, Urethra, and Rectum

Recommended Regimens

Cefixime 400 mg orally in a single dose,

OR

> **Ceftriaxone** 125 mg IM in a single dose,
>
> OR
>
> **Ciprofloxacin** 500 mg orally in a single dose,
>
> OR
>
> **Ofloxacin** 400 mg orally in a single dose,
>
> *PLUS*
>
> **Azithromycin** 1 g orally in a single dose,
>
> OR
>
> **Doxycycline** 100 mg orally twice a day for 7 days.

Cefixime has an antimicrobial spectrum similar to that of ceftriaxone, but the 400-mg oral dose does not provide as high nor as sustained a bactericidal level as that provided by the 125-mg dose of ceftriaxone. In published clinical trials, the 400-mg dose cured 97.1% of uncomplicated urogenital and anorectal gonococcal infections. The advantage of cefixime is that it can be administered orally.

Ceftriaxone in a single injection of 125 mg provides sustained, high bactericidal levels in the blood. Extensive clinical experience indicates that ceftriaxone is safe and effective for the treatment of uncomplicated gonorrhea at all sites, curing 99.1% of uncomplicated urogenital and anorectal infections in published clinical trials.

Ciprofloxacin is effective against most strains of *N. gonorrhoeae*. At a dose of 500 mg, ciprofloxacin provides sustained bactericidal levels in the blood; in published clinical trials, it has cured 99.8% of uncomplicated urogenital and anorectal infections. Ciprofloxacin is safe, relatively inexpensive, and can be administered orally.

Ofloxacin also is effective against most strains of *N. gonorrhoeae*, and it has favorable pharmacokinetics. The 400-mg oral dose has been effective for treatment of uncomplicated urogenital and anorectal infections, curing 98.4% of infections in published clinical trials.

Alternative Regimens

> **Spectinomycin** 2 g IM in a single dose. Spectinomycin is expensive and must be injected; however, it has been effective in published clinical trials, curing 98.2% of uncomplicated urogenital and anorectal gonococcal infections. Spectinomycin is useful for treatment of patients who cannot tolerate cephalosporins and quinolones.
>
> **Single-dose cephalosporin** regimens other than ceftriaxone 125 mg IM and cefixime 400 mg orally that are safe and highly effective against uncomplicated urogenital and anorectal gonococcal infections include a) ceftizoxime 500 mg IM, b) cefotaxime 500 mg IM, c) cefotetan 1 g IM, and d) cefoxitin 2 g IM with probenecid 1 g orally. None of these injectable cephalosporins offers any advantage in comparison with ceftriaxone, and clinical experience with these regimens for treatment of uncomplicated gonorrhea is limited.
>
> **Single-dose quinolone** regimens include enoxacin 400 mg orally, lomefloxacin 400 mg orally, and norfloxacin 800 mg orally. These regimens

appear to be safe and effective for the treatment of uncomplicated gonorrhea, but data regarding their use are limited. None of the regimens appears to offer any advantage over ciprofloxacin at a dose of 500 mg or ofloxacin at 400 mg.

Many other antimicrobials are active against *N. gonorrhoeae*; however, these guidelines are not intended to be a comprehensive list of all effective treatment regimens. Azithromycin 2 g orally is effective against uncomplicated gonococcal infection, but it is expensive and causes gastrointestinal distress too often to be recommended for treatment of gonorrhea. At an oral dose of 1 g, azithromycin is insufficiently effective, curing only 93% of patients in published studies.

Uncomplicated Gonococcal Infection of the Pharynx

Gonococcal infections of the pharynx are more difficult to eradicate than infections at urogenital and anorectal sites. Few antigonococcal regimens can reliably cure such infections >90% of the time.

Although chlamydial coinfection of the pharynx is unusual, coinfection at genital sites sometimes occurs. Therefore, treatment for both gonorrhea and chlamydia is suggested.

Recommended Regimens

Ceftriaxone 125 mg IM in a single dose,
OR
Ciprofloxacin 500 mg orally in a single dose,
OR
Ofloxacin 400 mg orally in a single dose,
PLUS
Azithromycin 1 g orally in a single dose,
OR
Doxycycline 100 mg orally twice a day for 7 days.

Follow-Up

Patients who have uncomplicated gonorrhea and who are treated with any of the recommended regimens need not return for a test of cure. Patients who have symptoms that persist after treatment should be evaluated by culture for *N. gonorrhoeae*, and any gonococci isolated should be tested for antimicrobial susceptibility. Infections identified after treatment with one of the recommended regimens usually result from reinfection rather than treatment failure, indicating a need for improved patient education and referral of sex partners. Persistent urethritis, cervicitis, or proctitis also may be caused by *C. trachomatis* and other organisms.

Management of Sex Partners

Patients should be instructed to refer sex partners for evaluation and treatment. All sex partners of patients who have *N. gonorrhoeae* infection should be evaluated and treated for *N. gonorrhoeae* and *C. trachomatis* infections if their last sexual contact with the patient was within 60 days before onset of symptoms or diagnosis of infection in the patient. If a patient's last sexual intercourse was >60 days before onset of symptoms or diagnosis, the patient's most recent sex partner should be treated. Patients should be instructed to avoid sexual intercourse until therapy is completed and they and their sex partners no longer have symptoms.

Special Considerations

Allergy, Intolerance, or Adverse Reactions

Persons who cannot tolerate cephalosporins or quinolones should be treated with spectinomycin. Because spectinomycin is unreliable (i.e., only 52% effective) against pharyngeal infections, patients who have suspected or known pharyngeal infection should have a pharyngeal culture evaluated 3–5 days after treatment to verify eradication of infection.

Pregnancy

Pregnant women should not be treated with quinolones or tetracyclines. Those infected with *N. gonorrhoeae* should be treated with a recommended or alternate cephalosporin. Women who cannot tolerate a cephalosporin should be administered a single 2-g dose of spectinomycin IM. Either erythromycin or amoxicillin is recommended for treatment of presumptive or diagnosed *C. trachomatis* infection during pregnancy (see Chlamydial Infection).

HIV Infection

Patients who have gonococcal infection and also are infected with HIV should receive the same treatment regimen as those who are HIV-negative.

Gonococcal Conjunctivitis

Only one study of the treatment of gonococcal conjunctivitis among adults in North America has been published recently. In that study, 12 of 12 patients responded favorably to a single 1-g IM injection of ceftriaxone. The following recommendations reflect the opinions of expert consultants.

Treatment

Recommended Regimen

Ceftriaxone 1 g IM in a single dose, and lavage the infected eye with saline solution once.

Management of Sex Partners

Patients should be instructed to refer their sex partners for evaluation and treatment (see Gonococcal Infection, Management of Sex Partners).

Disseminated Gonococcal Infection (DGI)

DGI results from gonococcal bacteremia. DGI often results in petechial or pustular acral skin lesions, asymmetrical arthralgia, tenosynovitis, or septic arthritis. The infection is complicated occasionally by perihepatitis, and rarely by endocarditis or meningitis. Strains of *N. gonorrhoeae* that cause DGI tend to cause minimal genital inflammation. In the United States, these strains have occurred infrequently during the past decade.

No studies of the treatment of DGI among persons in North America have been published recently. The following recommendations reflect the opinions of experts. No treatment failures have been reported.

Treatment

Hospitalization is recommended for initial therapy, especially for patients who cannot be relied on to comply with treatment, for those in whom the diagnosis is uncertain, and for those who have purulent synovial effusions or other complications. Patients should be examined for clinical evidence of endocarditis and meningitis. Patients treated for DGI should be treated presumptively for concurrent *C. trachomatis* infection unless appropriate testing excludes this infection.

Recommended Initial Regimen

Ceftriaxone 1 g IM or IV every 24 hours.

Alternative Initial Regimens

Cefotaxime 1 g IV every 8 hours,

OR

Ceftizoxime 1 g IV every 8 hours,

OR

For persons allergic to ß-lactam drugs:

Ciprofloxacin 500 mg IV every 12 hours,

OR

Ofloxacin 400 mg IV every 12 hours,

OR

Spectinomycin 2 g IM every 12 hours.

All regimens should be continued for 24–48 hours after improvement begins, at which time therapy may be switched to one of the following regimens to complete a full week of antimicrobial therapy:

Cefixime 400 mg orally twice a day,

OR

Ciprofloxacin 500 mg orally twice a day,

OR

Ofloxacin 400 mg orally twice a day.

Management of Sex Partners

Gonococcal infection often is asymptomatic in sex partners of patients who have DGI. As with uncomplicated gonococcal infections, patients should be instructed to refer their sex partners for evaluation and treatment (see Gonococcal Infection, Management of Sex Partners).

Gonococcal Meningitis and Endocarditis

Recommended Initial Regimen

Ceftriaxone 1–2 g IV every 12 hours.

Therapy for meningitis should be continued for 10–14 days; therapy for endo-carditis should be continued for at least 4 weeks. Treatment of complicated DGI should be undertaken in consultation with an expert.

Management of Sex Partners

Patients should be instructed to refer their sex partners for evaluation and treatment (see Gonococcal Infection, Management of Sex Partners).

Gonococcal Infection in Infants

Gonococcal infection usually results from exposure to infected cervical exudate at birth. It is usually an acute illness that becomes manifest 2–5 days after birth. The prevalence of infection among infants depends on the prevalence of infection among pregnant women, on whether pregnant women are screened for gonor-rhea, and on whether newborns receive ophthalmia prophylaxis.

The most serious manifestations of *N. gonorrhoeae* infection in newborns are ophthalmia neonatorum and sepsis, including arthritis and meningitis. Less serious manifestations include rhinitis, vaginitis, urethritis, and inflammation at sites of fetal monitoring.

Ophthalmia Neonatorum Caused by *N. gonorrhoeae*

Although *N. gonorrhoeae* is a less frequent cause of ophthalmia neonatorum in the United States than *C. trachomatis* and nonsexually transmitted agents, it is es-pecially important because it may result in perforation of the globe of the eye and in blindness.

Diagnostic Considerations

Infants at increased risk for gonococcal ophthalmia are those who do not receive ophthalmia prophylaxis and those whose mothers have had no prenatal care or whose mothers have a history of STDs or substance abuse. Gonococcal ophthalmia is strongly suggested when typical Gram-negative diplococci are iden-tified in conjunctival exudate, justifying presumptive treatment for gonorrhea after appropriate cultures for *N. gonorrhoeae* are obtained. Appropriate chlamydial test-ing should be done simultaneously. Presumptive treatment for *N. gonorrhoeae* may be indicated for newborns who are at increased risk for gonococcal ophthalmia and who have conjunctivitis but do not have gonococci in a Gram-stained smear of conjunctival exudate.

In all cases of neonatal conjunctivitis, conjunctival exudate should be cultured for *N. gonorrhoeae* and tested for antibiotic susceptibility before a definitive diag-nosis is made. A definitive diagnosis is important because of the public health and social consequences of a diagnosis of gonorrhea. Nongonococcal causes of neona-tal ophthalmia include *Moraxella catarrhalis* and other *Neisseria* species that are indistinguishable from *N. gonorrhoeae* on Gram-stained smear but can be differentiated in the microbiology laboratory.

Recommended Regimen

Ceftriaxone 25–50 mg/kg IV or IM in a single dose, not to exceed 125 mg.

NOTE: Topical antibiotic therapy alone is inadequate and is unnecessary if systemic treatment is administered.

Other Management Considerations

Simultaneous infection with *C. trachomatis* should be considered when a patient does not respond satisfactorily to treatment. Both mother and infant should be tested for chlamydial infection at the same time that gonorrhea testing is done (see Ophthalmia Neonatorum Caused by *C. trachomatis*). Ceftriaxone should be administered cautiously to hyperbilirubinemic infants, especially those born prematurely.

Follow-Up

Infants who have gonococcal ophthalmia should be hospitalized and evaluated for signs of disseminated infection (e.g., sepsis, arthritis, and meningitis). One dose of ceftriaxone is adequate therapy for gonococcal conjunctivitis, but many pediatricians prefer to continue antibiotics until cultures are negative at 48–72 hours. The duration of therapy should be decided in consultation with experienced physicians.

Management of Mothers and Their Sex Partners

The mothers of infants who have gonococcal infection and the mothers' sex partners should be evaluated and treated according to the recommendations for treating gonococcal infections in adults (see Gonococcal Infection in Adolescents and Adults).

Disseminated Gonococcal Infection and Gonococcal Scalp Abscess in Newborns

Sepsis, arthritis, meningitis, or any combination of these are rare complications of neonatal gonococcal infection. Localized gonococcal infection of the scalp might result from fetal monitoring through scalp electrodes. Detection of gonococcal infection in neonates who have sepsis, arthritis, meningitis, or scalp abscesses requires cultures of blood, CSF, and joint aspirate on chocolate agar. Specimens obtained from the conjunctiva, vagina, oropharynx, and rectum that are cultured on gonococcal selective medium are useful for identifying the primary site(s) of infection, especially if inflammation is present. Positive Gram-stained smears of exudate, CSF, or joint aspirate provide a presumptive basis for initiating treatment for *N. gonorrhoeae*. Diagnoses based on Gram-stained smears or presumptive identification of cultures should be confirmed with definitive tests on culture isolates.

Recommended Regimens

Ceftriaxone 25–50 mg/kg/day IV or IM in a single daily dose for 7 days, with a duration of 10–14 days if meningitis is documented;
OR
Cefotaxime 25 mg/kg IV or IM every 12 hours for 7 days, with a duration of 10–14 days if meningitis is documented.

Prophylactic Treatment for Infants Whose Mothers Have Gonococcal Infection

Infants born to mothers who have untreated gonorrhea are at high risk for infection.

Recommended Regimen in the Absence of Signs of Gonococcal Infection

---

Ceftriaxone 25–50 mg/kg IV or IM, not to exceed 125 mg, in a single dose.

Other Management Considerations

Mother and infant should be tested for chlamydial infection.

Follow-Up

A follow-up examination is not required.

Management of Mothers and Their Sex Partners

The mothers of infants who have gonococcal infection and the mothers' sex partners should be evaluated and treated according to the recommendations for treatment of gonococcal infections in adults (see Gonococcal Infection).

Gonococcal Infection in Children

After the neonatal period, sexual abuse is the most frequent cause of gonococcal infection in preadolescent children (see Sexual Assault or Abuse of Children). Vaginitis is the most common manifestation of gonococcal infection in preadolescent children. PID following vaginal infection is probably less common than among adults. Among sexually abused children, anorectal and pharyngeal infections with *N. gonorrhoeae* are common and frequently asymptomatic.

Diagnostic Considerations

Because of the legal implications of a diagnosis of *N. gonorrhoeae* infection in a child, only standard culture procedures for the isolation of *N. gonorrhoeae* should be used for children. Nonculture gonococcal tests for gonococci (e.g., Gram-stained smear, DNA probes, and EIA tests) should not be used alone; none of these tests have been approved by FDA for use with specimens obtained from the oropharynx, rectum, or genital tract of children. Specimens from the vagina, urethra, pharynx, or rectum should be streaked onto selective media for isolation of *N. gonorrhoeae*, and all presumptive isolates of *N. gonorrhoeae* should be identified definitively by at least two tests that involve different principles (e.g., biochemical, enzyme substrate, or serologic). Isolates should be preserved to enable additional or repeated testing.

Recommended Regimens for Children Who Weigh ≥45 kg

Children who weigh ≥45 kg should be treated with one of the regimens recommended for adults (see Gonococcal Infection).

NOTE: Quinolones are not approved for use in children because of concerns about toxicity based on animal studies. However, investigations of ciprofloxacin treatment in children who have cystic fibrosis demonstrated no adverse effects.

Recommended Regimen for Children Who Weigh <45 kg and Who Have Uncomplicated Gonococcal Vulvovaginitis, Cervicitis, Urethritis, Pharyngitis, or Proctitis

Ceftriaxone 125 mg IM in a single dose.

Alternative Regimen

Spectinomycin 40 mg/kg (maximum dose: 2 g) IM in a single dose may be used, but this therapy is unreliable for treatment of pharyngeal infections. Some experts use cefixime to treat gonococcal infections in children because it can be administered orally; however, no reports have been published concerning the safety or effectiveness of cefixime used for this purpose.

Recommended Regimen for Children Who Weigh <45 kg and Who Have Bacteremia or Arthritis

Ceftriaxone 50 mg/kg (maximum dose: 1 g) IM or IV in a single dose daily for 7 days.

Recommended Regimen for Children Who Weigh ≥45 kg and Who Have Bacteremia or Arthritis

Ceftriaxone 50 mg/kg (maximum dose: 2 g) IM or IV in a single dose daily for 10–14 days.

Follow-Up

Follow-up cultures are unnecessary if ceftriaxone is used. If spectinomycin is used to treat pharyngitis, a follow-up culture is necessary to ensure that treatment was effective.

Other Management Considerations

Only parenteral cephalosporins are recommended for use in children. Ceftriaxone is approved for all gonococcal infections in children; cefotaxime is approved for gonococcal ophthalmia only. Oral cephalosporins used for treatment of gonococcal infections in children have not been evaluated adequately.

All children who have gonococcal infections should be evaluated for coinfection with syphilis and *C. trachomatis.* For a discussion of concerns regarding sexual assault, refer to Sexual Assault or Abuse of Children.

Ophthalmia Neonatorum Prophylaxis

Instillation of a prophylactic agent into the eyes of all newborn infants is recommended to prevent gonococcal ophthalmia neonatorum; this procedure is required by law in most states. All the recommended prophylactic regimens in this section prevent gonococcal ophthalmia. However, the efficacy of these preparations in preventing chlamydial ophthalmia is less clear, and they do not eliminate nasopharyngeal colonization by *C. trachomatis.* The diagnosis and treatment of gonococcal and chlamydial infections in pregnant women is the best method for preventing neonatal gonococcal and chlamydial disease. Not all women, however, receive prenatal care; and ocular prophylaxis is warranted because it can prevent sight-threatening gonococcal ophthalmia and it is safe, easy to administer, and inexpensive.

Prophylaxis

Recommended Regimens

Silver nitrate (1%) aqueous solution in a single application,
OR
Erythromycin (0.5%) ophthalmic ointment in a single application,
OR
Tetracycline ophthalmic ointment (1%) in a single application.

One of these recommended preparations should be instilled into both eyes of every neonate as soon as possible after delivery. If prophylaxis is delayed (i.e., not administered in the delivery room), a monitoring system should be established to ensure that all infants receive prophylaxis. All infants should be administered ocular prophylaxis, regardless of whether delivery is vaginal or cesarian. Single-use tubes or ampules are preferable to multiple-use tubes. Bacitracin is not effective. Povidone iodine has not been studied adequately.

DISEASES CHARACTERIZED BY VAGINAL DISCHARGE

Management of Patients Who Have Vaginal Infections

Vaginitis is usually characterized by a vaginal discharge or vulvar itching and irritation; a vaginal odor may be present. The three diseases most frequently associated with vaginal discharge are trichomoniasis (caused by *T. vaginalis*), BV (caused by a replacement of the normal vaginal flora by an overgrowth of anaerobic microorganisms and *Gardnerella vaginalis*), and candidiasis (usually caused by *Candida albicans*). MPC caused by *C. trachomatis* or *N. gonorrhoeae* can sometimes cause vaginal discharge. Although vulvovaginal candidiasis usually is not transmitted sexually, it is included in this section because it is often diagnosed in women being evaluated for STDs.

Vaginitis is diagnosed by pH and microscopic examination of fresh samples of the discharge. The pH of the vaginal secretions can be determined by narrow-range pH paper for the elevated pH typical of BV or trichomoniasis (i.e., a pH of >4.5). One way to examine the discharge is to dilute a sample in one to two drops of 0.9% normal saline solution on one slide and 10% potassium hydroxide (KOH) solution on a second slide. An amine odor detected immediately after applying KOH suggests BV. A cover slip is placed on each slide, and they are examined under a microscope at low- and high-dry power. The motile *T. vaginalis* or the clue cells of BV usually are identified easily in the saline specimen. The yeast or pseudohyphae of *Candida* species are more easily identified in the KOH specimen. The presence of objective signs of vulvar inflammation in the absence of vaginal pathogens, along with a minimal amount of discharge, suggests the possibility of mechanical, chemical, allergic, or other noninfectious irritation of the vulva. Culture for *T. vaginalis* is more sensitive than microscopic examination. Laboratory testing fails to identify the cause of vaginitis among a substantial minority of women.

Bacterial Vaginosis

BV is a clinical syndrome resulting from replacement of the normal H_2O_2-producing *Lactobacillus* sp. in the vagina with high concentrations of anaerobic bacteria (e.g., *Prevotella* sp. and *Mobiluncus* sp.), *G. vaginalis*, and *Mycoplasma hominis*. BV is the most prevalent cause of vaginal discharge or malodor; however, half of the women whose illnesses meet the clinical criteria for BV are asymptomatic. The cause of the microbial alteration is not fully understood. Although BV is associated with having multiple sex partners, it is unclear whether BV results from acquisition of a sexually transmitted pathogen. Women who have never been sexually active are rarely affected. Treatment of the male sex partner has not been beneficial in preventing the recurrence of BV.

Diagnostic Considerations

BV can be diagnosed by the use of clinical or Gram stain criteria. Clinical criteria require three of the following symptoms or signs:

a. A homogeneous, white, noninflammatory discharge that smoothly coats the vaginal walls;
b. The presence of clue cells on microscopic examination;
c. A pH of vaginal fluid >4.5;
d. A fishy odor of vaginal discharge before or after addition of 10% KOH (i.e., the whiff test).

When a Gram stain is used, determining the relative concentration of the bacterial morphotypes characteristic of the altered flora of BV is an acceptable laboratory method for diagnosing BV. Culture of *G. vaginalis* is not recommended as a diagnostic tool because it is not specific.

Treatment

The principal goal of therapy for BV is to relieve vaginal symptoms and signs of infection. All women who have symptomatic disease require treatment, regardless of pregnancy status.

BV during pregnancy is associated with adverse pregnancy outcomes. The results of several investigations indicate that treatment of pregnant women who have BV and who are at high risk for preterm delivery (i.e., those who previously delivered a premature infant) might reduce the risk for prematurity. Therefore, high-risk pregnant women who do not have symptoms of BV may be evaluated for treatment.

Although some experts recommend treatment for high-risk pregnant women who have asymptomatic BV, others believe more information is needed before such a recommendation is made. A large, randomized clinical trial is underway to assess treatment for asymptomatic BV in pregnant women; the results of this investigation should clarify the benefits of therapy for BV in women at both low and high risk for preterm delivery.

The bacterial flora that characterizes BV has been recovered from the endometria and salpinges of women who have PID. BV has been associated with endometritis, PID, and vaginal cuff cellulitis after invasive procedures such as endometrial biopsy, hysterectomy, hysterosalpingography, placement of an intrauterine device, cesarean section, and uterine curettage. The results of one randomized controlled trial indicated that treatment of BV with metronidazole substantially reduced postabortion PID. On the basis of these data, consideration should be given to treatment of women who have symptomatic or asymptomatic BV before surgical abortion procedures are performed. However, more information is needed before recommending whether patients who have asymptomatic BV should be treated before other invasive procedures are performed.

Recommended Regimens for Nonpregnant Women

For treatment of pregnant women, see Bacterial Vaginosis, Special Considerations, Pregnancy.

Metronidazole 500 mg orally twice a day for 7 days,

OR

Clindamycin cream 2%, one full applicator (5 g) intravaginally at bedtime for 7 days,

OR

Metronidazole gel 0.75%, one full applicator (5 g) intravaginally twice a day for 5 days.

NOTE: Patients should be advised to avoid consuming alcohol during treatment with metronidazole and for 24 hours thereafter. Clindamycin cream is oil-based and might weaken latex condoms and diaphragms. Refer to condom product labeling for additional information.

Alternative Regimens

Metronidazole 2 g orally in a single dose,

OR

Clindamycin 300 mg orally twice a day for 7 days.

Metronidazole 2-g single-dose therapy is an alternative regimen because of its lower efficacy for BV. Oral metronidazole (500 mg twice a day) is efficacious for the treatment of BV, resulting in relief of symptoms and improvement in clinical course and flora disturbances. Based on efficacy data from four randomized controlled trials, overall cure rates 4 weeks after completion of treatment did not differ significantly between the 7-day regimen of oral metronidazole and the clindamycin vaginal cream (78% vs. 82%, respectively). Similarly, the results of another randomized controlled trial indicated that cure rates 7–10 days after completion of treatment did not differ significantly between the 7-day regimen of oral metronidazole and the metronidazole vaginal gel (84% vs. 75%, respectively). FDA has approved Flagyl ER[TM] (750 mg) once daily for 7 days for treatment of BV. However, data concerning clinical equivalency with other regimens have not been published.

Some health-care providers remain concerned about the possible teratogenicity of metronidazole, which has been suggested by experiments using extremely high and prolonged doses in animals. However, a recent meta-analysis does not indicate teratogenicity in humans. Some health-care providers prefer the intravaginal route because of a lack of systemic side effects (e.g., mild-to-moderate gastrointestinal disturbance and unpleasant taste). Mean peak serum concentrations of metronidazole after intravaginal administration are <2% the levels of standard 500-mg oral doses, and the mean bioavailability of clindamycin cream is approximately 4%.

Follow-Up

Follow-up visits are unnecessary if symptoms resolve. Recurrence of BV is not unusual. Because treatment of BV in high-risk pregnant women who are asymptomatic might prevent adverse pregnancy outcomes, a follow-up evaluation, at 1 month after completion of treatment, should be considered to evaluate whether therapy was successful. The alternative BV treatment regimens may be used to treat recurrent disease. No long-term maintenance regimen with any therapeutic agent is recommended.

Management of Sex Partners

The results of clinical trials indicate that a woman's response to therapy and the likelihood of relapse or recurrence are not affected by treatment of her sex partner(s). Therefore, routine treatment of sex partners is not recommended.

Special Considerations

Allergy or Intolerance to the Recommended Therapy

Clindamycin cream is preferred in case of allergy or intolerance to metronidazole. Metronidazole gel can be considered for patients who do not tolerate systemic metronidazole, but patients allergic to oral metronidazole should not be administered metronidazole vaginally.

Pregnancy

BV has been associated with adverse pregnancy outcomes (e.g., premature rupture of the membranes, preterm labor, and preterm birth), and the organisms found in increased concentration in BV also are frequently present in postpartum or postcesarean endometritis. Because treatment of BV in high-risk pregnant women (i.e., those who have previously delivered a premature infant) who are asymptomatic might reduce preterm delivery, such women may be screened, and those with BV can be treated. The screening and treatment should be conducted at the earliest part of the second trimester of pregnancy. The recommended regimen is metronidazole 250 mg orally three times a day for 7 days. The alternative regimens are a) metronidazole 2 g orally in a single dose or b) clindamycin 300 mg orally twice a day for 7 days.

Low-risk pregnant women (i.e., women who previously have not had a premature delivery) who have symptomatic BV should be treated to relieve symptoms. The recommended regimen is metronidazole 250 mg orally three times a day for 7 days. The alternative regimens are a) metronidazole 2 g orally in a single dose; b) clindamycin 300 mg orally twice a day for 7 days; or c) metronidazole gel, 0.75%, one full applicator (5 g) intravaginally, twice a day for 5 days. Some experts prefer the use of systemic therapy for low-risk pregnant women to treat possible subclinical upper genital tract infections.

Lower doses of medication are recommended for pregnant women to minimize exposure to the fetus. Data are limited concerning the use of metronidazole vaginal gel during pregnancy. The use of clindamycin vaginal cream during pregnancy is not recommended, because two randomized trials indicated an increase in the number of preterm deliveries among pregnant women who were treated with this medication.

HIV Infection

Patients who have BV and also are infected with HIV should receive the same treatment regimen as those who are HIV-negative.

Trichomoniasis

Trichomoniasis is caused by the protozoan *T. vaginalis*. Most men who are infected with *T. vaginalis* do not have symptoms of infection, although a minority of men have NGU. Many women do have symptoms of infection. Of these women, *T. vaginalis* characteristically causes a diffuse, malodorous, yellow-green discharge with vulvar irritation; many women have fewer symptoms. Vaginal trichomoniasis might be associated with adverse pregnancy outcomes, particularly premature rupture of the membranes and preterm delivery.

Recommended Regimen

Metronidazole 2 g orally in a single dose.

*Alternative Regimen**

Metronidazole 500 mg twice a day for 7 days.

Metronidazole is the only oral medication available in the United States for the treatment of trichomoniasis. In randomized clinical trials, the recommended metronidazole regimens have resulted in cure rates of approximately 90%–95%; ensuring treatment of sex partners might increase the cure rate. Treatment of patients and sex partners results in relief of symptoms, microbiologic cure, and reduction of transmission. Metronidazole gel is approved for treatment of BV, but, like other topically applied antimicrobials that are unlikely to achieve therapeutic levels in the urethra or perivaginal glands, it is considerably less efficacious for treatment of trichomoniasis than oral preparations of metronidazole and is not recommended for use. Several other topically applied antimicrobials have been used for treatment of trichomoniasis, but it is unlikely that these preparations will have greater efficacy than metronidazole gel.

Follow-Up

Follow-up is unnecessary for men and women who become asymptomatic after treatment or who are initially asymptomatic. Infections with strains of *T. vaginalis* that have diminished susceptibility to metronidazoie can occur; however, most of these organisms respond to higher doses of metronidazole. If treatment failure occurs with either regimen, the patient should be re-treated with metronidazole

---

*FDA has approved Flagyl 375™ mg twice a day for 7 days for treatment of trichomoniasis on the basis of pharmacokinetic equivalency of this regimen with metronidazole 250 mg three times a day for 7 days. No clinical data are available, however, to demonstrate clinical equivalency of the two regimens.

500 mg twice a day for 7 days. If treatment failure occurs repeatedly, the patient should be treated with a single 2-g dose of metronidazole once a day for 3–5 days.

Patients with culture-documented infection who do not respond to the regimens described in this report and in whom reinfection has been excluded should be managed in consultation with an expert; consultation is available from CDC. Evaluation of such cases should include determination of the susceptibility of *T. vaginalis* to metronidazole.

Management of Sex Partners

Sex partners should be treated. Patients should be instructed to avoid sex until they and their sex partners are cured. In the absence of a microbiologic test of cure, this means when therapy has been completed and patient and partner(s) are asymptomatic.

Special Considerations

Allergy, Intolerance, or Adverse Reactions

Effective alternatives to therapy with metronidazole are not available. Patients who are allergic to metronidazole can be managed by desensitization (*26*).

Pregnancy

Patients can be treated with 2 g of metronidazole in a single dose.

HIV Infection

Patients who have trichomoniasis and also are infected with HIV should receive the same treatment regimen as those who are HIV-negative.

Vulvovaginal Candidiasis

Vulvovaginal candidiasis (VVC) is caused by *C. albicans* or, occasionally, by other *Candida* sp., *Torulopsis* sp., or other yeasts. An estimated 75% of women will have at least one episode of VVC, and 40%–45% will have two or more episodes. A small percentage of women (i.e., probably <5%) experience recurrent VVC (RVVC). Typical symptoms of VVC include pruritus and vaginal discharge. Other symptoms may include vaginal soreness, vulvar burning, dyspareunia, and external dysuria. None of these symptoms is specific for VVC.

Diagnostic Considerations

A diagnosis of *Candida* vaginitis is suggested clinically by pruritus and erythema in the vulvovaginal area; a white discharge may occur. The diagnosis can be made in a woman who has signs and symptoms of vaginitis, and when either a) a wet preparation or Gram stain of vaginal discharge demonstrates yeasts or pseudohyphae or b) a culture or other test yields a positive result for a yeast species. *Candida* vaginitis is associated with a normal vaginal pH (≤4.5). Use of 10% KOH in wet preparations improves the visualization of yeast and mycelia by disrupting cellular material that might obscure the yeast or pseudohyphae. Identifying *Candida* by culture in the absence of symptoms should not lead to treatment, because approximately 10%–20% of women usually harbor *Candida* sp. and other yeasts in the vagina. VVC can occur concomitantly with STDs or frequently following antibacterial vaginal or systemic therapy.

Treatment

Topical formulations effectively treat VVC. The topically applied azole drugs are more effective than nystatin. Treatment with azoles results in relief of symptoms and negative cultures among 80%–90% of patients who complete therapy.

Recommended Regimens

Intravaginal agents:

Butoconazole 2% cream 5 g intravaginally for 3 days,*†

OR

Clotrimazole 1% cream 5 g intravaginally for 7–14 days,*†

OR

Clotrimazole 100 mg vaginal tablet for 7 days,*

OR

Clotrimazole 100 mg vaginal tablet, two tablets for 3 days,*

OR

Clotrimazole 500 mg vaginal tablet, one tablet in a single application,*

OR

Miconazole 2% cream 5 g intravaginally for 7 days,*†

OR

Miconazole 200 mg vaginal suppository, one suppository for 3 days,*†

OR

Miconazole 100 mg vaginal suppository, one suppository for 7 days,*†

OR

Nystatin 100,000-unit vaginal tablet, one tablet for 14 days,

OR

Tioconazole 6.5% ointment 5 g intravaginally in a single application,*†

OR

Terconazole 0.4% cream 5 g intravaginally for 7 days,*

OR

Terconazole 0.8% cream 5 g intravaginally for 3 days,*

OR

Terconazole 80 mg vaginal suppository, one suppository for 3 days.*

Oral agent:

Fluconazole 150 mg oral tablet, one tablet in single dose.

---

*These creams and suppositories are oil-based and might weaken latex condoms and diaphragms. Refer to condom product labeling for additional information.
†Over-the-counter (OTC) preparations.

Preparations for intravaginal administration of butaconazole, clotrimazole, miconazole, and tioconazole are available OTC, and women with VVC can choose one of those preparations. The duration for treatment with these preparations may be 1, 3, or 7 days. Self-medication with OTC preparations should be advised only for women who have been diagnosed previously with VVC and who have a recurrence of the same symptoms. Any woman whose symptoms persist after using an OTC preparation or who has a recurrence of symptoms within 2 months should seek medical care.

A new classification of VVC may facilitate antifungal selection as well as duration of therapy. Uncomplicated VVC (i.e., mild-to-moderate, sporadic, nonrecurrent disease in a normal host with normally susceptible *C. albicans*) responds to all the aforementioned azoles, even those that are short-term (<7 days) and single-dose therapies. In contrast, complicated VVC (i.e., severe local or recurrent VVC in an abnormal host [e.g., VVC in a patient who has uncontrolled diabetes, or infection caused by a less susceptible fungal pathogen such as *Candida glabrata*]) requires a longer duration of therapy (i.e, 10–14 days) with either topical or oral azoles. Additional studies confirming this approach are in progress.

Alternative Regimens

Several trials have demonstrated that oral azole agents (e.g., ketoconazole and itraconazole) might be as effective as topical agents. The ease of administering oral agents is an advantage over topical therapies. However, the potential for toxicity associated with using a systemic drug, particularly ketoconazole, must be considered.

Follow-Up

Patients should be instructed to return for follow-up visits only if symptoms persist or recur.

Management of Sex Partners

VVC usually is not acquired through sexual intercourse; treatment of sex partners is not recommended but may be considered for women who have recurrent infection. A minority of male sex partners may have balanitis, which is characterized by erythematous areas on the glans in conjunction with pruritus or irritation. These sex partners might benefit from treatment with topical antifungal agents to relieve symptoms.

Special Considerations

Allergy or Intolerance to the Recommended Therapy

Topical agents usually are free of systemic side effects, although local burning or irritation may occur. Oral agents occasionally cause nausea, abdominal pain, and headaches. Therapy with the oral azoles has been associated rarely with abnormal elevations of liver enzymes. Hepatotoxicity secondary to ketoconazole therapy occurs in an estimated one of every 10,000–15,000 exposed persons. Clinically important interactions might occur when these oral agents are administered with other drugs, including astemizole, calcium channel antagonists, cisapride, coumadin, cyclosporin A, oral hypoglycemic agents, phenytoin, protease inhibitors, tacrolimus, terfenadine, theophylline, trimetrexate, and rifampin.

Pregnancy

VVC often occurs during pregnancy. Only topical azole therapies should be used to treat pregnant women. Of those treatments that have been investigated for use during pregnancy, the most effective are butoconazole, clotrimazole, miconazole, and terconazole. Many experts recommend 7 days of therapy during pregnancy.

HIV Infection

Prospective controlled studies are in progress to confirm an alleged increase in incidence of VVC in HIV-infected women. No confirmed evidence has indicated a differential response to conventional antifungal therapy among HIV-positive women who have VVC. As such, women who have acute VVC and also are infected with HIV should receive the same treatment regimens as those who are HIV-negative.

Recurrent Vulvovaginal Candidiasis

RVVC, which usually is defined as *four* or more episodes of symptomatic VVC annually, affects a small percentage of women (i.e., probably <5%). The pathogenesis of RVVC is poorly understood. Risk factors for RVVC include uncontrolled diabetes mellitus, immunosuppression, and corticosteroid use. In some women who have RVVC, episodes occur after repeated courses of topical or systemic antibacterials. However, this association is not apparent in the majority of women. Most women who have RVVC have no apparent predisposing conditions. Clinical trials addressing the management of RVVC have involved continuing therapy between episodes.

Treatment

The optimal treatment for RVVC has not been established; however, an initial intensive regimen continued for approximately 10–14 days, followed immediately by a maintenance regimen for at least 6 months, is recommended. Maintenance ketoconazole 100 mg orally, once a day for ≤6 months, reduces the frequency of RVVC episodes. Investigations are evaluating a weekly fluconazole regimen, the results of which will be compared with once-monthly oral and topical antimycotic regimens that have only moderate protective efficacy. All cases of RVVC should be confirmed by culture before maintenance therapy is initiated.

Although patients with RVVC should be evaluated for predisposing conditions, routinely performing HIV testing for women with RVVC who do not have HIV risk factors is unnecessary.

Follow-Up

Patients who are receiving treatment for RVVC should receive regular follow-up evaluations to monitor the effectiveness of therapy and the occurrence of side effects.

Management of Sex Partners

Treatment of sex partners may be considered for partners who have symptomatic balanitis or penile dermatitis. However, routine treatment of sex partners usually is unnecessary.

Special Considerations

HIV Infection

Information is insufficient to determine the optimal management of RVVC among HIV-infected women. Until such information becomes available, management should be the same as for HIV-negative women who have RVVC.

PELVIC INFLAMMATORY DISEASE (PID)

PID comprises a spectrum of inflammatory disorders of the upper female genital tract, including any combination of endometritis, salpingitis, tubo-ovarian abscess, and pelvic peritonitis. Sexually transmitted organisms, especially *N. gonorrhoeae* and *C. trachomatis*, are implicated in most cases; however, microorganisms that can be part of the vaginal flora (e.g., anaerobes, *G. vaginalis, H. influenzae,* enteric Gram-negative rods, and *Streptococcus agalactiae*) also can cause PID. In addition, *M. hominis* and *U. urealyticum* might be etiologic agents of PID.

Diagnostic Considerations

Acute PID is difficult to diagnose because of the wide variation in the symptoms and signs. Many women with PID have subtle or mild symptoms that do not readily indicate PID. Consequently, delay in diagnosis and effective treatment probably contributes to inflammatory sequelae in the upper reproductive tract. Laparoscopy can be used to obtain a more accurate diagnosis of salpingitis and a more complete bacteriologic diagnosis. However, this diagnostic tool often is not readily available for acute cases, and its use is not easy to justify when symptoms are mild or vague. Moreover, laparoscopy will not detect endometritis and may not detect subtle inflammation of the fallopian tubes. Consequently, a diagnosis of PID usually is based on clinical findings.

The clinical diagnosis of acute PID also is imprecise. Data indicate that a clinical diagnosis of symptomatic PID has a PPV for salpingitis of 65%–90% in comparison with laparoscopy. The PPV of a clinical diagnosis of acute PID differs depending on epidemiologic characteristics and the clinical setting, with higher PPV among sexually active young (especially teenaged) women and among patients attending STD clinics or from settings in which rates of gonorrhea or chlamydia are high. In all settings, however, no single historical, physical, or laboratory finding is both sensitive and specific for the diagnosis of acute PID (i.e., can be used both to detect all cases of PID and to exclude all women without PID). Combinations of diagnostic findings that improve either sensitivity (i.e., detect more women who have PID) or specificity (i.e., exclude more women who do not have PID) do so only at the expense of the other. For example, requiring two or more findings excludes more women who do not have PID but also reduces the number of women with PID who are identified.

Many episodes of PID go unrecognized. Although some cases are asymptomatic, others are undiagnosed because the patient or the health-care provider fails to recognize the implications of mild or nonspecific symptoms or signs (e.g., abnormal bleeding, dyspareunia, or vaginal discharge [atypical PID]). Because of the difficulty of diagnosis and the potential for damage to the reproductive health of women even by apparently mild or atypical PID, health-care providers should maintain a low threshold for the diagnosis of PID. Even so, the long-term outcome of early treatment of women with asymptomatic or atypical PID is unknown. The following recommendations for diagnosing PID are intended to help health-care providers recognize when PID should be suspected and when they need to obtain additional information to increase diagnostic certainty. These recommendations are based partially on the fact that diagnosis and management of other common causes of lower abdominal pain (e.g., ectopic pregnancy, acute appendicitis, and functional pain) are unlikely to be impaired by initiating empiric antimicrobial therapy for PID.

Empiric treatment of PID should be initiated in sexually active young women and others at risk for STDs if all the following **minimum criteria** are present and no other cause(s) for the illness can be identified:

- Lower abdominal tenderness,

- Adnexal tenderness, and

- Cervical motion tenderness.

More elaborate diagnostic evaluation often is needed, because incorrect diagnosis and management might cause unnecessary morbidity. These additional criteria may be used to enhance the specificity of the minimum criteria listed previously. **Additional criteria** that support a diagnosis of PID include the following:

- Oral temperature >101 F (>38.3 C),

- Abnormal cervical or vaginal discharge,

- Elevated erythrocyte sedimentation rate,

- Elevated C-reactive protein, and

- Laboratory documentation of cervical infection with *N. gonorrhoeae* or *C. trachomatis.*

The **definitive criteria** for diagnosing PID, which are warranted in selected cases, include the following:

- Histopathologic evidence of endometritis on endometrial biopsy,

- Transvaginal sonography or other imaging techniques showing thickened fluid-filled tubes with or without free pelvic fluid or tubo-ovarian complex, and

- Laparoscopic abnormalities consistent with PID.

Although treatment can be initiated before bacteriologic diagnosis of *C. trachomatis* or *N. gonorrhoeae* infection, such a diagnosis emphasizes the need to treat sex partners.

Treatment

PID treatment regimens must provide empiric, broad-spectrum coverage of likely pathogens. Antimicrobial coverage should include *N. gonorrhoeae, C. trachomatis*, anaerobes, Gram-negative facultative bacteria, and streptococci. Although several antimicrobial regimens have been effective in achieving a clinical and microbiologic cure in randomized clinical trials with short-term follow-up, few investigations have a) assessed and compared these regimens with regard to elimination of infection in the endometrium and fallopian tubes or b) determined the incidence of long-term complications (e.g., tubal infertility and ectopic pregnancy).

All regimens should be effective against *N. gonorrhoeae* and *C. trachomatis,* because negative endocervical screening does not preclude upper-reproductive tract infection. Although the need to eradicate anaerobes from women who have PID has not been determined definitively, the evidence suggests that this may be important. Anaerobic bacteria have been isolated from the upper-reproductive tract of women who have PID, and data from in vitro studies have revealed that anaerobes such as *Bacteroides fragilis* can cause tubal and epithelial destruction. In addition, BV also is diagnosed in many women who have PID. Until treatment regimens that do not adequately cover these microbes have been shown to prevent sequelae as well as the regimens that are effective against these microbes, the recommended regimens should have anaerobic coverage. Treatment should be initiated as soon as the presumptive diagnosis has been made, because prevention of long-term sequelae has been linked directly with immediate administration of appropriate antibiotics. When selecting a treatment regimen, health-care providers should consider availability, cost, patient acceptance, and antimicrobial susceptibility.

In the past, many experts recommended that all patients who had PID be hospitalized so that bed rest and supervised treatment with parenteral antibiotics could be initiated. However, hospitalization is no longer synonymous with parenteral therapy. No currently available data compare the efficacy of parenteral with oral therapy or inpatient with outpatient treatment settings. Until the results from ongoing trials comparing parenteral inpatient therapy with oral outpatient therapy for women who have mild PID are available, such decisions must be based on observational data and consensus opinion. The decision of whether hospitalization is necessary should be based on the discretion of the health-care provider.

The following criteria for **HOSPITALIZATION** are based on observational data and theoretical concerns:

- Surgical emergencies such as appendicitis cannot be excluded;

- The patient is pregnant;

- The patient does not respond clinically to oral antimicrobial therapy;

- The patient is unable to follow or tolerate an outpatient oral regimen;

- The patient has severe illness, nausea and vomiting, or high fever;

- The patient has a tubo-ovarian abscess; or

- The patient is immunodeficient (i.e., has HIV infection with low CD4 counts, is taking immunosuppressive therapy, or has another disease).

Most clinicians favor at least 24 hours of direct inpatient observation for patients who have tubo-ovarian abscesses, after which time home parenteral therapy should be adequate.

There are no efficacy data comparing parenteral with oral regimens. Experts have extensive experience with both of the following regimens. Also, there are multiple randomized trials demonstrating the efficacy of each regimen. Although most trials have used parenteral treatment for at least 48 hours after the patient demonstrates substantial clinical improvement, this is an arbitrary designation. Clinical experience should guide decisions regarding transition to oral therapy, which may be accomplished within 24 hours of clinical improvement.

Parenteral Regimen A

Cefotetan 2 g IV every 12 hours,

OR

Cefoxitin 2 g IV every 6 hours,

PLUS

Doxycycline 100 mg IV or orally every 12 hours.

NOTE: Because of pain associated with infusion, doxycycline should be administered orally when possible, even when the patient is hospitalized. Both oral and IV administration of doxycycline provide similar bioavailability. In the event that IV administration is necessary, use of lidocaine or other short-acting local anesthetic, heparin, or steroids with a steel needle or extension of the infusion time may reduce infusion complications. Parenteral therapy may be discontinued 24 hours after a patient improves clinically, and oral therapy with doxycycline (100 mg twice a day) should continue for a total of 14 days. When tubo-ovarian abscess is present, many health-care providers use clindamycin or metronidazole with doxycycline for continued therapy rather than doxycycline alone, because it provides more effective anaerobic coverage.

Clinical data are limited regarding the use of other second- or third-generation cephalosporins (e.g., ceftizoxime, cefotaxime, and ceftriaxone), which also might be effective therapy for PID and might replace cefotetan or cefoxitin. However, they are less active than cefotetan or cefoxitin against anaerobic bacteria.

Parenteral Regimen B

Clindamycin 900 mg IV every 8 hours,
> **PLUS**

Gentamicin loading dose IV or IM (2 mg/kg of body weight), followed by a maintenance dose (1.5 mg/kg) every 8 hours. Single daily dosing may be substituted.

NOTE: Although use of a single daily dose of gentamicin has not been evaluated for the treatment of PID, it is efficacious in other analogous situations. Parenteral therapy may be discontinued 24 hours after a patient improves clinically, and continuing oral therapy should consist of doxycycline 100 mg orally twice a day or clindamycin 450 mg orally four times a day to complete a total of 14 days of therapy. When tubo-ovarian abscess is present, many health-care providers use clindamycin for continued therapy rather than doxycycline, because clindamycin provides more effective anaerobic coverage.

Alternative Parenteral Regimens

Limited data support the use of other parenteral regimens, but the following three regimens have been investigated in at least one clinical trial, and they have broad spectrum coverage.

Ofloxacin 400 mg IV every 12 hours,
> **PLUS**

Metronidazole 500 mg IV every 8 hours.
> **OR**

Ampicillin/Sulbactam 3 g IV every 6 hours,
> **PLUS**

Doxycycline 100 mg IV or orally every 12 hours.
> **OR**

Ciprofloxacin 200 mg IV every 12 hours,
> **PLUS**

Doxycycline 100 mg IV or orally every 12 hours,
> **PLUS**

Metronidazole 500 mg IV every 8 hours.

Ampicillin/sulbactam plus doxycycline has good coverage against *C. trachomatis, N. gonorrhoeae*, and anaerobes and appears to be effective for patients who have tubo-ovarian abscess. Both IV ofloxacin and ciprofloxacin have been investigated as single agents. Because ciprofloxacin has poor coverage against *C. trachomatis*, it is recommended that doxycycline be added routinely. Because of concerns regarding the anaerobic coverage of both quinolones, metronidazole should be included with each regimen.

Oral Treatment

As with parenteral regimens, clinical trials of outpatient regimens have provided minimal information regarding intermediate and long-term outcomes. The following regimens provide coverage against the frequent etiologic agents of PID, but evidence from clinical trials supporting their use is limited. Patients who do not respond to oral therapy within 72 hours should be reevaluated to confirm the diagnosis and be administered parenteral therapy on either an outpatient or inpatient basis.

Regimen A

Ofloxacin 400 mg orally twice a day for 14 days,
PLUS
Metronidazole 500 mg orally twice a day for 14 days.

Oral ofloxacin has been investigated as a single agent in two well-designed clinical trials, and it is effective against both *N. gonorrhoeae and C. trachomatis.* Despite the results of these trials, ofloxacin's lack of anaerobic coverage is a concern; the addition of metronidazole provides this coverage.

Regimen B

Ceftriaxone 250 mg IM once,
OR
Cefoxitin 2 g IM plus **Probenecid** 1 g orally in a single dose concurrently once,
OR
Other parenteral third-generation **cephalosporin** (e.g., **ceftizoxime** or **cefotaxime**),
PLUS
Doxycycline 100 mg orally twice a day for 14 days. (Include this regimen with one of the above regimens.)

The optimal choice of a cephalosporin for Regimen B is unclear; although cefoxitin has better anaerobic coverage, ceftriaxone has better coverage against *N. gonorrhoeae.* Clinical trials have demonstrated that a single dose of cefoxitin is effective in obtaining short-term clinical response in women who have PID; however, the theoretical limitations in its coverage of anaerobes may require the addition of metronidazole. The metronidazole also will effectively treat BV, which also is frequently associated with PID. No data have been published regarding the use of oral cephalosporins for the treatment of PID.

Alternative Oral Regimens

Information regarding other outpatient regimens is limited, but one other regimen has undergone at least one clinical trial and has broad spectrum coverage. Amoxicillin/clavulanic acid plus doxycycline was effective in obtaining short-term clinical response in a single clinical trial; however, gastrointestinal symptoms might limit the overall success of this regimen. Several recent investigations have evaluated the use of azithromycin in the treatment of upper-reproductive tract infections; however, the data are insufficient to recommend this agent as a component of any of the treatment regimens for PID.

Follow-Up

Patients receiving oral or parenteral therapy should demonstrate substantial clinical improvement (e.g., defervescence; reduction in direct or rebound abdominal tenderness; and reduction in uterine, adnexal, and cervical motion tenderness) within 3 days after initiation of therapy. Patients who do not demonstrate improvement within this time period usually require additional diagnostic tests, surgical intervention, or both.

If the health-care provider prescribes outpatient oral or parenteral therapy, a follow-up examination should be performed within 72 hours, using the criteria for clinical improvement described previously. Some experts also recommend rescreening for *C. trachomatis* and *N. gonorrhoeae* 4–6 weeks after therapy is completed. If PCR or LCR is used to document a test of cure, rescreening should be delayed for 1 month after completion of therapy.

Management of Sex Partners

Sex partners of patients who have PID should be examined and treated if they had sexual contact with the patient during the 60 days preceding onset of symptoms in the patient. The evaluation and treatment are imperative because of the risk for reinfection and the strong likelihood of urethral gonococcal or chlamydial infection in the sex partner. Male partners of women who have PID caused by *C. trachomatis* and/or *N. gonorrhoeae* often are asymptomatic.

Sex partners should be treated empirically with regimens effective against both of these infections, regardless of the apparent etiology of PID or pathogens isolated from the infected woman.

Even in clinical settings in which only women are treated, special arrangements should be made to provide care for male sex partners of women who have PID. When this is not feasible, health-care providers should ensure that sex partners are referred for appropriate treatment.

Special Considerations

Pregnancy

Because of the high risk for maternal morbidity, fetal wastage, and preterm delivery, pregnant women who have suspected PID should be hospitalized and treated with parenteral antibiotics.

HIV Infection

Differences in the clinical manifestations of PID between HIV-infected women and HIV-negative women have not been well delineated. In early observational studies, HIV-infected women with PID were more likely to require surgical intervention. In a subsequent and more comprehensive observational study, HIV-infected women who had PID had more severe symptoms than HIV-negative women but responded equally well to standard parenteral antibiotic regimens. In another study, the microbiologic findings for HIV-infected and HIV-negative women were similar, except for higher rates of concomitant *Candida* and HPV infections and HPV-related cytologic abnormalities among HIV-infected women. Immunosuppressed HIV-infected women who have PID should be managed aggressively using one of the parenteral antimicrobial regimens recommended in this report.

EPIDIDYMITIS

Among sexually active men aged <35 years, epididymitis is most often caused by *C. trachomatis* or *N. gonorrhoeae*. Epididymitis caused by sexually transmitted *E. coli* infection also occurs among homosexual men who are the insertive partners during anal intercourse. Sexually transmitted epididymitis usually is accompanied by urethritis, which often is asymptomatic. Nonsexually transmitted epididymitis associated with urinary tract infections caused by Gram-negative enteric organisms occurs more frequently among men aged >35 years, men who have recently undergone urinary tract instrumentation or surgery, and men who have anatomical abnormalities.

Although most patients can be treated on an outpatient basis, hospitalization should be considered when severe pain suggests other diagnoses (e.g., torsion, testicular infarction, and abscess) or when patients are febrile or might be noncompliant with an antimicrobial regimen.

Diagnostic Considerations

Men who have epididymitis typically have unilateral testicular pain and tenderness; hydrocele and palpable swelling of the epididymis usually are present. Testicular torsion, a surgical emergency, should be considered in all cases but is more frequent among adolescents. Torsion occurs more frequently in patients who do not have evidence of inflammation or infection. Emergency testing for torsion may be indicated when the onset of pain is sudden, pain is severe, or the test results available during the initial examination do not enable a diagnosis of urethritis or urinary tract infection to be made. If the diagnosis is questionable, an expert should be consulted immediately, because testicular viability may be compromised. The evaluation of men for epididymitis should include the following procedures:

- A Gram-stained smear of urethral exudate or intraurethral swab specimen for diagnosis of urethritis (i.e., ≥5 polymorphonuclear leukocytes per oil immersion field) and for presumptive diagnosis of gonococcal infection.

- A culture of urethral exudate or intraurethral swab specimen, or nucleic acid amplification test (either on intraurethral swab or first-void urine) for *N. gonorrhoeae* and *C. trachomatis*.

- Examination of first-void urine for leukocytes if the urethral Gram stain is negative. Culture and Gram-stained smear of uncentrifuged urine should be obtained.

- Syphilis serology and HIV counseling and testing.

Treatment

Empiric therapy is indicated before culture results are available. Treatment of epididymitis caused by *C. trachomatis* or *N. gonorrhoeae* will result in a) a microbiologic cure of infection, b) improvement of the signs and symptoms, c) prevention of transmission to others, and d) a decrease in the potential complications (e.g., infertility or chronic pain).

Recommended Regimens

For epididymitis most likely caused by gonococcal or chlamydial infection:
> **Ceftriaxone** 250 mg IM in a single dose,
> > ***PLUS***
> **Doxycycline** 100 mg orally twice a day for 10 days.

For epididymitis most likely caused by enteric organisms, or for patients allergic to cephalosporins and/or tetracyclines:
> **Ofloxacin** 300 mg orally twice a day for 10 days.

As an adjunct to therapy, bed rest, scrotal elevation, and analgesics are recommended until fever and local inflammation have subsided.

Follow-Up

Failure to improve within 3 days requires reevaluation of both the diagnosis and therapy. Swelling and tenderness that persist after completion of antimicrobial therapy should be evaluated comprehensively. The differential diagnosis includes tumor, abscess, infarction, testicular cancer, and tuberculous or fungal epididymitis.

Management of Sex Partners

Patients who have epididymitis that is known or suspected to be caused by *N. gonorrhoeae* or *C. trachomatis* should be instructed to refer sex partners for evaluation and treatment. Sex partners of these patients should be referred if their contact with the index patient was within the 60 days preceding onset of symptoms in the patient.

Patients should be instructed to avoid sexual intercourse until they and their sex partners are cured. In the absence of a microbiologic test of cure, this means until therapy is completed and patient and partner(s) no longer have symptoms.

Special Considerations

HIV Infection

Patients who have uncomplicated epididymitis and also are infected with HIV should receive the same treatment regimen as those who are HIV-negative. Fungi and mycobacteria, however, are more likely to cause epididymitis in immunosuppressed patients than in immunocompetent patients.

HUMAN PAPILLOMAVIRUS INFECTION

Genital Warts

More than 20 types of HPV can infect the genital tract. Most HPV infections are asymptomatic, subclinical, or unrecognized. Visible genital warts usually are caused by HPV types 6 or 11. Other HPV types in the anogenital region (i.e., types 16, 18, 31, 33, and 35) have been strongly associated with cervical dysplasia. Diagnosis of genital warts can be confirmed by biopsy, although biopsy is rarely needed (e.g., if the diagnosis is uncertain; the lesions do not respond to standard therapy; the disease worsens during therapy; the patient is immunocompromised; or warts are pigmented, indurated, fixed, and ulcerated). No data support the use of type-specific HPV nucleic acid tests in the routine diagnosis or management of visible genital warts.

HPV types 6 and 11 also can cause warts on the uterine cervix and in the vagina, urethra, and anus; these warts are sometimes symptomatic. Intra-anal warts are seen predominately in patients who have had receptive anal intercourse; these warts are distinct from perianal warts, which can occur in men and women who do not have a history of anal sex. Other than the genital area, these HPV types have been associated with conjunctival, nasal, oral, and laryngeal warts. HPV types 6 and 11 are associated rarely with invasive squamous cell carcinoma of the external genitalia. Depending on the size and anatomic locations, genital warts can be painful, friable, and/or pruritic.

HPV types 16, 18, 31, 33, and 35 are found occasionally in visible genital warts and have been associated with external genital (i.e., vulvar, penile, and anal) squamous intraepithelial neoplasia (i.e., squamous cell carcinoma in situ, bowenoid papulosis, Erythroplasia of Queyrat, or Bowen's disease of the genitalia). These HPV types have been associated with vaginal, anal, and cervical intraepithelial dysplasia and squamous cell carcinoma. Patients who have visible genital warts can be infected simultaneously with multiple HPV types.

Treatment

The primary goal of treating visible genital warts is the removal of symptomatic warts. Treatment can induce wart-free periods in most patients. Genital warts often are asymptomatic. No evidence indicates that currently available treatments eradicate or affect the natural history of HPV infection. The removal of warts may or may not decrease infectivity. If left untreated, visible genital warts may resolve on their own, remain unchanged, or increase in size or number. No evidence indicates that treatment of visible warts affects the development of cervical cancer.

Regimens

Treatment of genital warts should be guided by the preference of the patient, the available resources, and the experience of the health-care provider. None of the available treatments is superior to other treatments, and no single treatment is ideal for all patients or all warts.

The available treatments for visible genital warts are patient-applied therapies (i.e., podofilox and imiquimod) and provider-administered therapies (i.e., cryotherapy, podophyllin resin, trichloroacetic acid [TCA], bichloroacetic acid [BCA], interferon, and surgery). Most patients have from one to 10 genital warts, with a total wart area of 0.5–1.0 cm^2, that are responsive to most treatment modalities. Factors that might influence selection of treatment include wart size, wart number, anatomic site of wart, wart morphology, patient preference, cost of treatment, convenience, adverse effects, and provider experience. Having a treatment plan or protocol is important, because many patients will require a course of therapy rather than a single treatment. In general, warts located on moist surfaces and/or in intertriginous areas respond better to topical treatment (e.g., TCA, podophyllin, podofilox, and imiquimod) than do warts on drier surfaces.

The treatment modality should be changed if a patient has not improved substantially after three provider-administered treatments or if warts have not completely cleared after six treatments. The risk-benefit ratio of treatment should be evaluated throughout the course of therapy to avoid overtreatment. Providers should be knowledgeable about, and have available to them, at least one patient-applied and one provider-administered treatment.

Complications rarely occur if treatments for warts are employed properly. Patients should be warned that scarring in the form of persistent hypopigmentation or hyperpigmentation is common with ablative modalities. Depressed or hypertrophic scars are rare but can occur, especially if the patient has had insufficient time to heal between treatments. Treatment can result rarely in disabling chronic pain syndromes (e.g., vulvodynia or hyperesthesia of the treatment site).

External Genital Warts, Recommended Treatments

Patient-Applied:

Podofilox 0.5% solution or gel. Patients may apply podofilox solution with a cotton swab, or podofilox gel with a finger, to visible genital warts twice a day for 3 days, followed by 4 days of no therapy. This cycle may be repeated as necessary for a total of four cycles. The total wart area treated should not exceed 10 cm^2, and a total volume of podofilox should not exceed 0.5 mL per day. If possible, the health-care provider should apply the initial treatment to demonstrate the proper application technique and identify which warts should be treated. *The safety of podofilox during pregnancy has not been established.*

OR

Imiquimod 5% cream. Patients should apply imiquimod cream with a finger at bedtime, three times a week for as long as 16 weeks. The treatment area should be washed with mild soap and water 6–10 hours after the application. Many patients may be clear of warts by 8–10 weeks or sooner. *The safety of imiquimod during pregnancy has not been established.*

Provider-Administered:

Cryotherapy with liquid nitrogen or cryoprobe. Repeat applications every 1 to 2 weeks.

OR

Podophyllin resin 10%–25% in compound tincture of benzoin. A small amount should be applied to each wart and allowed to air dry. To avoid the possibility of complications associated with systemic absorption and toxicity, some experts recommend that application be limited to ≤0.5 mL of podophyllin or ≤10 cm^2 of warts per session. Some experts suggest that the preparation should be thoroughly washed off 1–4 hours after application to reduce local irritation. Repeat weekly if necessary. *The safety of podophyllin during pregnancy has not been established.*

OR

TCA or BCA 80%–90%. Apply a small amount only to warts and allow to dry, at which time a white "frosting" develops; powder with talc or sodium bicarbonate (i.e., baking soda) to remove unreacted acid if an excess amount is applied. Repeat weekly if necessary.

OR

Surgical removal either by tangential scissor excision, tangential shave excision, curettage, or electrosurgery.

External Genital Warts, Alternative Treatments

Intralesional interferon,

OR

Laser surgery.

For patient-applied treatments, patients must be able to identify and reach warts to be treated. Podofilox 0.5% solution or gel is relatively inexpensive, easy to use, safe, and self-applied by patients. Podofilox is an antimitotic drug that results in destruction of warts. Most patients experience mild/moderate pain or local irritation after treatment. Imiquimod is a topically active immune enhancer that stimulates production of interferon and other cytokines. Before wart resolution, local inflammatory reactions are common; these reactions usually are mild to moderate.

Cryotherapy, which requires the use of basic equipment, destroys warts by thermal-induced cytolysis. Its major drawback is that proper use requires substantial training, without which warts are frequently overtreated or undertreated, resulting in poor efficacy or increased likelihood of complications. Pain after application of the liquid nitrogen, followed by necrosis and sometimes blistering, are not unusual. Although local anesthesia (topical or injected) is not used routinely, its use facilitates treatment if there are many warts or if the area of warts is large.

Podophyllin resin contains a number of compounds, including the podophyllin lignans that are antimitotic. The resin is most frequently compounded at 10%–25% in tincture of benzoin. However, podophyllin resin preparations differ in the concentration of active components and contaminants. The shelf life and stability of podophyllin preparations are unknown. It is important to apply a thin layer of podophyllin resin to the warts and allow it to air dry before the treated area comes into contact with clothing. Overapplication or failure to air dry can result in local irritation caused by spread of the compound to adjacent areas.

Both TCA and BCA are caustic agents that destroy warts by chemical coagulation of the proteins. Although these preparations are widely used, they have not been investigated thoroughly. TCA solutions have a low viscosity comparable to water and can spread rapidly if applied excessively, thus damaging adjacent normal tissue. Both TCA and BCA should be applied sparingly and allowed to dry before the patient sits or stands. If pain is intense, the acid can be neutralized with soap or sodium bicarbonate (i.e., baking soda).

Surgical removal of warts has an advantage over other treatment modalities in that it renders the patient wart-free, usually with a single visit. However, substantial clinical training, additional equipment, and a longer office visit are required. Once local anesthesia is achieved, the visible genital warts can be physically destroyed by electrosurgery, in which case no additional hemostasis is required. Alternatively, the warts can be removed either by tangential excision with a pair of fine scissors or a scalpel or by curettage. Because most warts are exophytic, this can be accomplished with a resulting wound that only extends into the upper dermis. Hemostasis can be achieved with an electrosurgical unit or a chemical styptic (e.g., an aluminum chloride solution). Suturing is neither required nor indicated in most cases when surgical removal is done properly. Surgery is most beneficial for patients who have a large number or area of genital warts. Carbon dioxide laser and surgery may be useful in the management of extensive warts or intraurethral warts, particularly for those patients who have not responded to other treatments.

Interferons, either natural or recombinant, used for the treatment of genital warts have been administered systemically (i.e., subcutaneously at a distant site or IM) and intralesionally (i.e., injected into the warts). Systemic interferon is not effective. The efficacy and recurrence rates of intralesional interferon are comparable to other treatment modalities. Interferon is believed to be effective because of antiviral and/or immunostimulating effects. However, interferon therapy is not recommended for routine use because of inconvenient routes of administration, frequent office visits, and the association between its use and a high frequency of systemic adverse effects.

Because of the shortcomings of available treatments, some clinics employ combination therapy (i.e., the simultaneous use of two or more modalities on the same wart at the same time). Most experts believe that combining modalities does not increase efficacy but may increase complications.

Cervical Warts

For women who have exophytic cervical warts, high-grade squamous intraepithelial lesions (SIL) must be excluded before treatment is begun. Management of exophytic cervical warts should include consultation with an expert.

Vaginal Warts

Cryotherapy with liquid nitrogen. The use of a cryoprobe in the vagina is not recommended because of the risk for vaginal perforation and fistula formation.

OR

TCA or BCA 80%–90% applied only to warts. Apply a small amount only to warts and allow to dry, at which time a white "frosting" develops; powder with talc or sodium bicarbonate (i.e., baking soda) to remove unreacted acid if an excess amount is applied. Repeat weekly if necessary.

OR

Podophyllin 10%–25% in compound tincture of benzoin applied to a treated area that must be dry before the speculum is removed. Treat with ≤2 cm^2 per session. Repeat application at weekly intervals. Because of concern about potential systemic absorption, some experts caution against vaginal application of podophyllin. *The safety of podophyllin during pregnancy has not been established.*

Urethral Meatus Warts

Cryotherapy with liquid nitrogen,

OR

Podophyllin 10%–25% in compound tincture of benzoin. The treatment area must be dry before contact with normal mucosa. Podophyllin must be applied weekly if necessary. *The safety of podophyllin during pregnancy has not been established.*

Anal Warts

Cryotherapy with liquid nitrogen.

OR

TCA or BCA 80%–90% applied to warts. Apply a small amount only to warts and allow to dry, at which time a white "frosting" develops; powder with talc or sodium bicarbonate (i.e., baking soda) to remove unreacted acid if an excess amount is applied. Repeat weekly if necessary.

OR

Surgical removal.

Note: Management of warts on rectal mucosa should be referred to an expert.

Oral Warts

Cryotherapy with liquid nitrogen,

OR

Surgical removal.

Follow-Up

After visible genital warts have cleared, a follow-up evaluation is not mandatory. Patients should be cautioned to watch for recurrences, which occur most frequently during the first 3 months. Because the sensitivity and specificity of self-diagnosis of genital warts is unknown, patients concerned about recurrences should be offered a follow-up evaluation 3 months after treatment. Earlier follow-up visits also may be useful a) to document a wart-free state, b) to monitor for or treat complications of therapy, and c) to provide the opportunity for patient education and counseling. Women should be counseled regarding the need for regular cytologic screening as recommended for women without genital warts. The presence of genital warts is not an indication for cervical colposcopy.

Management of Sex Partners

Examination of sex partners is not necessary for the management of genital warts because the role of reinfection is probably minimal and, in the absence of curative therapy, treatment to reduce transmission is not realistic. However, because self- or partner-examination has not been evaluated as a diagnostic method for genital warts, sex partners of patients who have genital warts may benefit from examination to assess the presence of genital warts and other STDs. Sex partners also might benefit from counseling about the implications of having a partner who has genital warts. Because treatment of genital warts probably does not eliminate the HPV infection, patients and sex partners should be cautioned that the patient might remain infectious even though the warts are gone. The use of condoms may reduce, but does not eliminate, the risk for transmission to uninfected partners. Female sex partners of patients who have genital warts should be reminded that cytologic screening for cervical cancer is recommended for all sexually active women.

Special Considerations

Pregnancy

Imiquimod, podophyllin, and podofilox should not be used during pregnancy. Because genital warts can proliferate and become friable during pregnancy, many experts advocate their removal during pregnancy. HPV types 6 and 11 can cause laryngeal papillomatosis in infants and children. The route of transmission (i.e., transplacental, perinatal, or postnatal) is not completely understood. The preventive value of cesarean section is unknown; thus, cesarean delivery should not be performed solely to prevent transmission of HPV infection to the newborn. In rare

94

instances, cesarean delivery may be indicated for women with genital warts if the pelvic outlet is obstructed or if vaginal delivery would result in excessive bleeding.

Immunosuppressed Patients

Persons who are immunosuppressed because of HIV or other reasons may not respond as well as immunocompetent persons to therapy for genital warts, and they may have more frequent recurrences after treatment. Squamous cell carcinomas arising in or resembling genital warts might occur more frequently among immunosuppressed persons, requiring more frequent biopsy for confirmation of diagnosis.

Squamous Cell Carcinoma in situ

Patients in whom squamous cell carcinoma in situ of the genitalia is diagnosed should be referred to an expert for treatment. Ablative modalities usually are effective, but careful follow-up is important. The risk for these lesions leading to invasive squamous cell carcinoma of the external genitalia in immunocompetent patients is unknown but is probably low. Female partners of patients who have squamous cell carcinoma in situ are at high risk for cervical abnormalities.

Subclinical Genital HPV Infection (Without Exophytic Warts)

Subclinical genital HPV infection occurs more frequently than visible genital warts among both men and women. Infection often is indirectly diagnosed on the cervix by Pap smear, colposcopy, or biopsy and on the penis, vulva, and other genital skin by the appearance of white areas after application of acetic acid. However, the routine use of acetic acid soaks and examination with light and magnification, as a screening test, to detect "subclinical" or "acetowhite" genital warts is not recommended. Acetowhitening is not a specific test for HPV infection. Thus, in populations at low risk for this infection, many false-positives may be detected when this test is used for screening. The specificity and sensitivity of this procedure has not been defined. In special situations, experienced clinicians find this test useful for identification of flat genital warts.

A definitive diagnosis of HPV infection depends on detection of viral nucleic acid (DNA or RNA) or capsid protein. Pap smear diagnosis of HPV does not always correlate with detection of HPV DNA in cervical cells. Cell changes attributed to HPV in the cervix are similar to those of mild dysplasia and often regress spontaneously without treatment. Tests that detect several types of HPV DNA or RNA in cells scraped from the cervix are available, but the clinical utility of these tests for managing patients is unclear. Management decisions should not be made on the basis of HPV tests. Screening for subclinical genital HPV infection using DNA or RNA tests or acetic acid is not recommended.

Treatment

In the absence of coexistent dysplasia, treatment is not recommended for subclinical genital HPV infection diagnosed by Pap smear, colposcopy, biopsy, acetic acid soaking of genital skin or mucous membranes, or the detection of HPV (DNA or RNA). The diagnosis of subclinical genital HPV infection is often questionable, and no therapy has been identified to eradicate infection. HPV has been demonstrated in adjacent tissue after laser treatment of HPV-associated dysplasia and after attempts to eliminate subclinical HPV by extensive laser vaporization of the anogenital area. In the presence of coexistent dysplasia, management should be based on the grade of dysplasia.

Management of Sex Partners

Examination of sex partners is unnecessary. Most sex partners of infected patients probably are already infected subclinically with HPV. No practical screening tests for subclinical infection are available. The use of condoms may reduce transmission to sex partners who are likely to be uninfected (e.g., new partners); however, the period of communicability is unknown. Whether patients who have subclinical HPV infection are as contagious as patients who have exophytic warts is unknown.

CERVICAL CANCER SCREENING FOR WOMEN WHO ATTEND STD CLINICS OR HAVE A HISTORY OF STDs

Women who have a history of STD are at increased risk for cervical cancer, and women attending STD clinics may have other risk factors that place them at even greater risk. Prevalence studies have determined that precursor lesions for cervical cancer occur about five times more frequently among women attending STD clinics than among women attending family planning clinics.

The Pap smear (i.e., cervical smear) is an effective and relatively low-cost screening test for invasive cervical cancer and SIL,* the precursors of cervical cancer. Both ACOG and the American Cancer Society (ACS) recommend annual Pap smears for all sexually active women. Although these guidelines take the position that Pap smears can be obtained less frequently in some situations, women with a history of STDs may need more frequent screening because of their increased risk for cervical cancer. Moreover, surveys of women attending STD clinics indicate that many women do not understand the purpose or importance of Pap smears, and almost half of the women who have had a pelvic examination erroneously believe they have had a Pap smear when they actually have not.

---

*The *1988 Bethesda System for Reporting Cervical/Vaginal Cytologic Diagnoses* introduced the terms "low-grade SIL" and "high-grade SIL" (*27*). Low-grade SIL encompasses cellular changes associated with HPV and mild dysplasia/cervical intraepithelial neoplasia 1 (CIN 1). High-grade SIL includes moderate dysplasia/CIN 2, severe dysplasia/CIN 3, and carcinoma in situ/CIN 3.

Recommendations

At the time of a pelvic examination for STD screening, the health-care provider should inquire about the result of the patient's last Pap smear and discuss the following information with the patient:

- The purpose and importance of a Pap smear;

- Whether a Pap smear was obtained during the clinic visit;

- The need for an annual Pap smear; and

- The names of local providers or referral clinics that can obtain Pap smears and adequately follow up results (i.e., if a Pap smear was not obtained during this examination).

If a woman has not had a Pap smear during the previous 12 months, a Pap smear should be obtained as part of the routine pelvic examination. Health-care providers should be aware that, after a pelvic examination, many women believe they have had a Pap smear when they actually have not, and thus may report having had a recent Pap smear. Therefore, in STD clinics, a Pap smear should be strongly considered during the routine clinical evaluation of women who have not had a normal Pap smear within the preceding 12 months that is documented within the clinic record or linked-system record.

A woman may benefit from receiving printed information about Pap smears and a report containing a statement that a Pap smear was obtained during her clinic visit. If possible, a copy of the Pap smear result should be provided to the patient for her records.

Follow-Up

Clinics and health-care providers who provide Pap smear screening services are encouraged to use cytopathology laboratories that report results using the Bethesda System of classification. If the results of the Pap smear are abnormal, care should be provided according to the *Interim Guidelines for Management of Abnormal Cervical Cytology* published by the National Cancer Institute Consensus Panel and briefly summarized below (*27*). Appropriate follow-up of Pap smears showing a high-grade SIL always includes referral to a clinician who has the capacity to provide a colposcopic examination of the lower genital tract and, if indicated, colposcopically directed biopsies. For a Pap smear showing low-grade SIL or atypical squamous cells of undetermined significance (ASCUS), follow-up without colposcopy *may* be acceptable in circumstances when the diagnosis is not qualified further or the cytopathologist favors a reactive process. In general, this would involve repeated Pap smears every 4–6 months for 2 years until the results of three consecutive smears have been negative. If repeated smears show persistent abnormalities, colposcopy and directed biopsy are indicated for low-grade SIL and should be considered for ASCUS. Women with a diagnosis of unqualified ASCUS associated with severe inflammation should at least be reevaluated with a repeat Pap smear after 2–3 months, then repeated Pap smears every 4–6 months for

2 years until the results of three consecutive smears have been negative. If specific infections are identified, the patient should be reevaluated after appropriate treatment for those infections. In all follow-up strategies using repeated Pap smears, the tests not only must be negative but also must be interpreted by the laboratory as "satisfactory for evaluation."

Because many public health clinics, including most STD clinics, cannot provide clinical follow-up of abnormal Pap smears with colposcopy and biopsy, women with Pap smears demonstrating high grade SIL or persistent low-grade SIL or ASCUS usually will need a referral to other local health-care providers or clinics for colposcopy and biopsy. Clinics and health-care providers who offer Pap smear screening services but cannot provide appropriate colposcopic follow-up of abnormal Pap smears should arrange referral services that a) can promptly evaluate and treat patients and b) will report the results of the evaluation to the referring clinician or health-care provider. Clinics and health-care providers should develop protocols that identify women who miss initial appointments (i.e., so that these women can be scheduled for repeat Pap smears), and they should reevaluate such protocols routinely. Pap smear results, type and location of follow-up appointments, and results of follow-up should be clearly documented in the clinic record. The development of colposcopy and biopsy services in local health departments, especially in circumstances where referrals are difficult and follow-up is unlikely, should be considered.

Other Management Considerations

Other considerations in performing Pap smears are as follows:

- The Pap smear is not an effective screening test for STDs.

- If a woman is menstruating, a Pap smear should be postponed, and the woman should be advised to have a Pap smear at the earliest opportunity.

- The presence of a mucopurulent discharge might compromise interpretation of the Pap smear. However, if the woman is unlikely to return for follow-up, a Pap smear can be obtained after careful removal of the discharge with a saline-soaked cotton swab.

- A woman who has external genital warts does not need to have Pap smears more frequently than a woman who does not have warts, unless otherwise indicated.

- In an STD clinic setting or when other cultures or specimens are collected for STD diagnoses, the Pap smear may be obtained last.

- Women who have had a hysterectomy do not require an annual Pap smear unless the hysterectomy was related to cervical cancer or its precursor lesions. In this situation, women should be advised to continue follow-up with the physician(s) who provided health care at the time of the hysterectomy.

- Both health-care providers who receive basic retraining on Pap smear collection and clinics that use simple quality assurance measures obtain fewer unsatisfactory smears.

- Although type-specific HPV testing to identify women at high and low risk for cervical cancer may become clinically relevant in the future, its utility in clinical practice is unclear, and such testing is not recommended.

Special Considerations

Pregnancy

Women who are pregnant should have a Pap smear as part of routine prenatal care. A cytobrush may be used for obtaining Pap smears in pregnant women, although care should be taken not to disrupt the mucous plug.

HIV Infection

Several studies have documented an increased prevalence of SIL in HIV-infected women, and HIV is believed by many experts to hasten the progression of precursor lesions to invasive cervical cancer. The following recommendations for Pap smear screening among HIV-infected women are consistent with other guidelines published by the U.S. Department of Health and Human Services (10,11,27,28) and are based partially on the opinions of experts in the care and management of cervical cancer and HIV infection in women.

- After obtaining a complete history of previous cervical disease, HIV-infected women should have a comprehensive gynecologic examination, including a pelvic examination and Pap smear as part of their initial evaluation. A Pap smear should be obtained twice in the first year after diagnosis of HIV infection and, if the results are normal, annually thereafter. If the results of the Pap smear are abnormal, care should be provided according to the *Interim Guidelines for Management of Abnormal Cervical Cytology* (*28*). Women who have a cytological diagnosis of high-grade SIL or squamous cell carcinoma should undergo colposcopy and directed biopsy. HIV infection is not an indication for colposcopy in women who have normal Pap smears.

VACCINE-PREVENTABLE STDs

One of the most effective means of preventing the transmission of STDs is preexposure immunization. Currently licensed vaccines for the prevention of STDs include those for hepatitis A and hepatitis B. Clinical development and trials are underway for vaccines against a number of other STDs, including HIV and HSV. As more vaccines become available, immunization possibly will become one of the most widespread methods used to prevent STDs.

Five different viruses (i.e., hepatitis A–E) account for almost all cases of viral hepatitis in humans. Serologic testing is necessary to confirm the diagnosis. For example, a health-care provider might assume that an injecting-drug user with jaundice has hepatitis B when, in fact, outbreaks of hepatitis A among injecting-drug users often occur. The correct diagnosis is essential for the delivery of appropriate preventive services. To ensure accurate reporting of viral hepatitis and appropriate prophylaxis of household contacts and sex partners, all case reports of viral hepatitis should be investigated and the etiology established through serologic testing.

Hepatitis A

Hepatitis A is caused by infection with the hepatitis A virus (HAV). HAV replicates in the liver and is shed in the feces. Virus in the stool is found in the highest concentrations from 2 weeks before to 1 week after the onset of clinical illness. Virus also is present in serum and saliva during this period, although in much lower concentrations than in feces. The most common mode of HAV transmission is fecal-oral, either by person-to-person transmission between household contacts or sex partners or by contaminated food or water. Because viremia occurs in acute infection, bloodborne HAV transmission can occur; however, such cases have been reported infrequently. Although HAV is present in low concentrations in the saliva of infected persons, no evidence indicates that saliva is involved in transmission.

Of patients who have acute hepatitis A, ≤20% require hospitalization; fulminant liver failure develops in 0.1% of patients. The overall mortality rate for acute hepatitis A is 0.3%, but it is higher (1.8%) for adults aged >49 years. HAV infection is not associated with chronic liver disease.

In the United States during 1995, 31,582 cases of hepatitis A were reported. The most frequently reported source of infection was household or sexual contact with a person who had hepatitis A, followed by attendance or employment at a day care center; recent international travel; homosexual activity; injecting-drug use; and a suspected food or waterborne outbreak. Many persons who have hepatitis A do not identify risk factors; their source of infection may be other infected persons who are asymptomatic. The prevalence of previous HAV infection among the U.S. population is 33% (CDC, unpublished data).

Outbreaks of hepatitis A among homosexual men have been reported in urban areas, both in the United States and in foreign countries. In one investigation, the prevalence of HAV infection among homosexual men was significantly higher (30%) than that among heterosexual men (12%). In New York City, a case-control study of homosexual men who had acute hepatitis A determined that case-patients were more likely to have had more anonymous sex partners and to have engaged in group sex than were the control subjects; oral-anal intercourse (i.e., the oral role) and digital-rectal intercourse (i.e., the digital role) also were associated with illness.

Treatment

Because HAV infection is self-limited and does not result in chronic infection or chronic liver disease, treatment is usually supportive. Hospitalization may be necessary for patients who are dehydrated because of nausea and vomiting or who have fulminant hepatitis A. Medications that might cause liver damage or that are metabolized by the liver should be used with caution. No specific diet or activity restrictions are necessary.

Prevention

General measures for hepatitis A prevention (e.g., maintenance of good personal hygiene) have not been successful in interrupting outbreaks of hepatitis A when the mode of transmission is from person to person, including sexual contact. To help control hepatitis A outbreaks among homosexual and bisexual men, health education messages should stress the modes of HAV transmission and the measures that can be taken to reduce the risk for transmission of any STD, including enterically transmitted agents such as HAV. However, vaccination is the most effective means of preventing HAV infection.

Two types of products are available for the prevention of hepatitis A: immune globulin (IG) and hepatitis A vaccine. IG is a solution of antibodies prepared from human plasma that is made with a serial ethanol precipitation procedure that inactivates HBV and HIV. When administered intramuscularly before exposure to HAV, or within 2 weeks after exposure, IG is >85% effective in preventing hepatitis A. IG administration is recommended for a variety of exposure situations (e.g., for persons who have sexual or household contact with patients who have hepatitis A). The duration of protection is relatively short (i.e., 3–6 months) and dose dependent.

Inactivated hepatitis A vaccines have been available in the United States since 1995. These vaccines, administered as a two-dose series, are safe, highly immunogenic, and efficacious. Immunogenicity studies indicate that 99%–100% of persons respond to one dose of hepatitis A vaccine; the second dose provides long-term protection. Efficacy studies indicate that inactivated hepatitis A vaccines are 94%–100% effective in preventing HAV infection (2).

Preexposure Prophylaxis

Vaccination with hepatitis A vaccine for preexposure protection against HAV infection is indicated for persons who have the following risk factors and who are likely to seek treatment in settings where STDs are being treated.

- **Men who have sex with men.** Sexually active men who have sex with men (both adolescents and adults) should be vaccinated.

- **Illegal drug users.** Vaccination is recommended for users of illegal injecting and noninjecting drugs if local epidemiologic evidence indicates previous or current outbreaks among persons with such risk behaviors.

Postexposure Prophylaxis

Persons who were exposed recently to HAV (i.e., household or sexual contact with a person who has hepatitis A) and who had not been vaccinated before the exposure should be administered a single IM dose of IG (0.02 mL/kg) as soon as possible, but not >2 weeks after exposure. Persons who received at least one dose of hepatitis A vaccine ≥1 month before exposure to HAV do not need IG.

Hepatitis B

Hepatitis B is a common STD. During the past 10 years, sexual transmission accounted for approximately 30%–60% of the estimated 240,000 new HBV infections that occurred annually in the United States. Chronic HBV infection develops in 1%–6% of persons infected as adults. These persons are capable of transmitting HBV to others, and they are at risk for chronic liver disease. In the United States, HBV infection leads to an estimated 6,000 deaths annually; these deaths result from cirrhosis of the liver and primary hepatocellular carcinoma.

The risk for perinatal HBV infection among infants born to HBV-infected mothers is 10%–85%, depending on the mother's hepatitis B e antigen (HbeAg) status. Chronic HBV infection develops in approximately 90% of infected newborns; these children are at high risk for chronic liver disease. Even when not infected during the perinatal period, children of HBV-infected mothers are at high risk for acquiring chronic HBV infection by person-to-person transmission during the first 5 years of life.

Treatment

No specific treatment is available for persons who have acute HBV infection. Supportive and symptomatic care usually are the mainstays of therapy. During the past decade, numerous antiviral agents have been investigated for treatment of chronic HBV infection. Alpha-2b interferon has been 40% effective in eliminating chronic HBV infection; persons who became infected during adulthood were most likely to respond to this treatment. Antiretroviral agents (e.g., lamivudine) have been effective in eliminating HBV infection, and a number of other compounds are being evaluated. The goal of antiviral treatment is to stop HBV replication. Response to treatment can be demonstrated by normalization of liver function tests, improvement in liver histology, and seroreversion from HBeAg-positive to HBeAg-negative. Long-term follow-up of treated patients suggests that the remission of chronic hepatitis induced by alpha interferon is of long duration. Patient characteristics associated with positive response to interferon therapy include low pretherapy HBV DNA levels, high pretherapy alanine aminotransferase levels, short duration of infection, acquisition of disease in adulthood, active histology, and female sex.

Prevention

Although methods used to prevent other STDs should prevent HBV infection, hepatitis B vaccination is the most effective means of preventing infection. The epidemiology of HBV infection in the United States indicates that multiple age groups must be targeted to provide widespread immunity and effectively prevent HBV transmission and HBV-related chronic liver disease (1). Vaccination of persons who have a history of STDs is part of a comprehensive strategy to eliminate HBV transmission in the United States. This comprehensive strategy also includes prevention of perinatal HBV infection by a) routine screening of all pregnant women, b) routine vaccination of all newborns, c) vaccination of older children at high risk for HBV infection (e.g., Alaskan Natives, Pacific Islanders, and residents in households of first-generation immigrants from countries in which HBV is of high or intermediate endemicity), d) vaccination of children aged 11–12 years who have not previously received hepatitis B vaccine, and e) vaccination of adolescents and adults at high risk for infection.

Preexposure Prophylaxis

With the implementation of routine infant hepatitis B vaccination and the wide-scale implementation of vaccination programs for adolescents, vaccination of adults at high risk for HBV has become a priority in the strategy to eliminate HBV transmission in the United States. All persons attending STD clinics and persons known to be at high risk for HBV infection (e.g., persons with multiple sex partners, sex partners of persons with chronic HBV infection, and injecting-drug users) should be offered hepatitis B vaccine and advised of their risk for HBV infection (as well as their risk for HIV infection) and the means to reduce their risk (i.e., exclusivity in sexual relationships, use of condoms, and avoidance of nonsterile drug-injection equipment).

Persons who should receive hepatitis B vaccine include the following:

- Sexually active homosexual and bisexual men;

- Sexually active heterosexual men and women, including those a) in whom another STD was recently diagnosed, b) who had more than one sex partner in the preceding 6 months, c) who received treatment in an STD clinic, and d) who are prostitutes;

- Illegal drug users, including injecting-drug users and users of illegal noninjecting drugs;

- Health-care workers;

- Recipients of certain blood products;

- Household and sexual contacts of persons who have chronic HBV infection;

- Adoptees from countries in which HBV infection is endemic;

- Certain international travelers;

- Clients and employees of facilities for the developmentally disabled;

- Infants and children; and

- Hemodialysis patients.

Screening for Antibody Versus Vaccination Without Screening

The prevalence of previous HBV infection among sexually active homosexual men and among injecting-drug users is high. Serologic screening for evidence of previous infection before vaccinating adult members of these groups may be cost-effective, depending on the costs of laboratory testing and vaccine. At the current cost of vaccine, prevaccination testing on adolescents is not cost-effective. For adults attending STD clinics, the prevalence of HBV infection and the vaccine cost may justify prevaccination testing. However, because prevaccination testing may lower compliance with vaccination, the first dose of vaccine should be administered at the time of testing. The additional doses of hepatitis vaccine should be administered on the basis of the prevaccination test results. The preferred serologic test for prevaccination testing is the total antibody to hepatitis B core antigen (anti-HBc), because it will detect persons who have either resolved or chronic infection. Because anti-HBc testing will not identify persons immune to HBV infection as a result of vaccination, a history of hepatitis B vaccination should be obtained, and fully vaccinated persons should not be revaccinated.

Vaccination Schedules

Hepatitis B vaccine is highly immunogenic. Protective levels of antibody are present in approximately 50% of young adults after one dose of vaccine; in 85%, after two doses; and >90%, after three doses. The third dose is required to provide long-term immunity. The most often used schedule is vaccination at 0, 1–2, and 4–6 months. The first and second doses of vaccine must be administered at least 1 month apart, and the first and third doses at least 4 months apart. If the vaccination series is interrupted after the first or second dose of vaccine, the missing dose should be administered as soon as possible. The series should not be restarted if a dose has been missed. The vaccine should be administered IM in the deltoid, not in the buttock.

Postexposure Prophylaxis

Exposure to Persons Who Have Acute Hepatitis B

Sexual Contacts

Patients who have acute HBV infection are potentially infectious to persons with whom they have sexual contact. Passive immunization with hepatitis B immune globulin (HBIG) prevents 75% of these infections. Hepatitis B vaccination alone is less effective in preventing infection than HBIG and vaccination. Sexual contacts of patients who have acute hepatitis B should receive HBIG and begin the hepatitis B vaccine series within 14 days after the most recent sexual contact. Testing of sex partners for susceptibility to HBV infection (anti-HBc) can be considered if it does not delay treatment >14 days.

Nonsexual Household Contacts

Nonsexual household contacts of patients who have acute hepatitis B are not at high risk for infection unless they are exposed to the patient's blood (e.g., by sharing a toothbrush or razor blade). However, vaccination of household contacts is encouraged, especially for children and adolescents. If the patient remains HBsAg-positive after 6 months (i.e., becomes chronically infected), all household contacts should be vaccinated.

Exposure to Persons Who Have Chronic HBV Infection

Hepatitis B vaccination without the use of HBIG is highly effective in preventing HBV infection in household and sexual contacts of persons who have chronic HBV infection, and all such contacts should be vaccinated. Postvaccination serologic testing is indicated for sex partners of persons who have chronic hepatitis B infections and for infants born to HBsAg-positive women.

Special Considerations

Pregnancy

Pregnancy is not a contraindication to hepatitis B vaccine or HBIG vaccine administration.

HIV Infection

HBV infection in HIV-infected persons is more likely to lead to chronic HBV infection. HIV infection also can impair the response to hepatitis B vaccine. Therefore, HIV-infected persons who are vaccinated should be tested for hepatitis B surface antibody 1–2 months after the third vaccine dose. Revaccination with three more doses should be considered for those who do not respond initially to vaccination. Those who do not respond to additional doses should be advised that they might remain susceptible to HBV infection.

PROCTITIS, PROCTOCOLITIS, AND ENTERITIS

Sexually transmitted gastrointestinal syndromes include proctitis, proctocolitis, and enteritis. Proctitis occurs predominantly among persons who participate in anal intercourse, and enteritis occurs among those whose sexual practices include oral-fecal contact. Proctocolitis can be acquired by either route, depending on the pathogen. Evaluation should include appropriate diagnostic procedures (e.g., anoscopy or sigmoidoscopy, stool examination, and culture).

Proctitis is an inflammation limited to the rectum (the distal 10–12 cm) that is associated with anorectal pain, tenesmus, and rectal discharge. *N. gonorrhoeae*, *C. trachomatis* (including LGV serovars), *T. pallidum*, and HSV usually are the sexually transmitted pathogens involved. In patients coinfected with HIV, herpes proctitis may be especially severe.

Proctocolitis is associated with symptoms of proctitis plus diarrhea and/or abdominal cramps and inflammation of the colonic mucosa extending to 12 cm. Fecal leukocytes may be detected on stool examination depending on the pathogen. Pathogenic organisms include *Campylobacter* sp., *Shigella* sp., *Entamoeba histolytica*, and, rarely, *C. trachomatis* (LGV serovars). CMV or other opportunistic agents may be involved in immunosuppressed HIV-infected patients.

Enteritis usually results in diarrhea and abdominal cramping without signs of proctitis or proctocolitis. In otherwise healthy patients, *Giardia lamblia* is most frequently implicated. Among HIV-infected patients, other infections that usually are not sexually transmitted may occur, including CMV, *Mycobacterium avium-intracellulare*, *Salmonella* sp., *Cryptosporidium*, *Microsporidium*, and *Isospora*. Multiple stool examinations may be necessary to detect *Giardia*, and special stool preparations are required to diagnose cryptosporidiosis and microsporidiosis. Additionally, enteritis may be a primary effect of HIV infection.

When laboratory diagnostic capabilities are available, treatment should be based on the specific diagnosis. Diagnostic and treatment recommendations for all enteric infections are beyond the scope of these guidelines.

Treatment

Acute proctitis of recent onset among persons who have recently practiced receptive anal intercourse is most often sexually transmitted. Such patients should be examined by anoscopy and should be evaluated for infection with HSV, *N. gonorrhoeae*, *C. trachomatis*, and *T. pallidum*. If anorectal pus is found on examination, or if polymorphonuclear leukocytes are found on a Gram-stained smear of anorectal secretions, the following therapy may be prescribed pending results of additional laboratory tests.

Recommended Regimen

Ceftriaxone 125 mg IM (or another agent effective against anal and genital gonorrhea),

PLUS

Doxycycline 100 mg orally twice a day for 7 days.

NOTE: For patients who have herpes proctitis, refer to Genital Herpes Simplex Virus (HSV) Infection.

Follow-Up

Follow-up should be based on specific etiology and severity of clinical symptoms. Reinfection may be difficult to distinguish from treatment failure.

Management of Sex Partners

Sex partners of patients who have sexually transmitted enteric infections should be evaluated for any diseases diagnosed in the patient.

ECTOPARASITIC INFECTIONS

Pediculosis Pubis

Patients who have pediculosis pubis (i.e., pubic lice) usually seek medical attention because of pruritus. Such patients also usually notice lice or nits on their pubic hair.

Recommended Regimens

Permethrin 1% creme rinse applied to affected areas and washed off after 10 minutes.

OR

> **Lindane** 1% shampoo applied for 4 minutes to the affected area, and then thoroughly washed off. This regimen is not recommended for pregnant or lactating women or for children aged <2 years.
> **OR**
> **Pyrethrins with piperonyl butoxide** applied to the affected area and washed off after 10 minutes.

The lindane regimen is the least expensive therapy; toxicity, as indicated by seizure and aplastic anemia, has not been reported when treatment was limited to the recommended 4-minute period. Permethrin has less potential for toxicity than lindane.

Other Management Considerations

The recommended regimens should not be applied to the eyes. Pediculosis of the eyelashes should be treated by applying occlusive ophthalmic ointment to the eyelid margins twice a day for 10 days.

Bedding and clothing should be decontaminated (i.e., either machine-washed or machine-dried using the heat cycle or dry-cleaned) or removed from body contact for at least 72 hours. Fumigation of living areas is not necessary.

Follow-Up

Patients should be evaluated after 1 week if symptoms persist. Re-treatment may be necessary if lice are found or if eggs are observed at the hair-skin junction. Patients who do not respond to one of the recommended regimens should be retreated with an alternative regimen.

Management of Sex Partners

Sex partners within the preceding month should be treated.

Special Considerations

Pregnancy

Pregnant and lactating women should be treated with either permethrin or pyrethrins with piperonyl butoxide.

HIV Infection

Patients who have pediculosis pubis and also are infected with HIV should receive the same treatment regimen as those who are HIV-negative.

Scabies

The predominant symptom of scabies is pruritus. Sensitization to *Sarcoptes scabiei* must occur before pruritus begins. The first time a person is infected with *S. scabiei*, sensitization takes several weeks to develop. Pruritus might occur within 24 hours after a subsequent reinfestation. Scabies in adults may be sexually transmitted, although scabies in children usually is not.

Recommended Regimen

Permethrin cream (5%) applied to all areas of the body from the neck down and washed off after 8–14 hours.

Alternative Regimens

Lindane (1%) 1 oz. of lotion or 30 g of cream applied thinly to all areas of the body from the neck down and thoroughly washed off after 8 hours.

OR

Sulfur (6%) precipitated in ointment applied thinly to all areas nightly for 3 nights. Previous applications should be washed off before new applications are applied. Thoroughly wash off 24 hours after the last application.

Permethrin is effective and safe but costs more than lindane. Lindane is effective in most areas of the country, but lindane resistance has been reported in some areas of the world, including parts of the United States. Seizures have occurred when lindane was applied after a bath or used by patients who had extensive dermatitis. Aplastic anemia following lindane use also has been reported.

NOTE: Lindane should not be used after a bath, and it should not be used by a) persons who have extensive dermatitis, b) pregnant or lactating women, and c) children aged <2 years.

Ivermectin (single oral dose of 200 µg/kg or 0.8% topical solution) is a potential new therapeutic modality. However, no controlled clinical trials have been conducted to compare ivermectin with the currently recommended therapies.

Other Management Considerations

Bedding and clothing should be decontaminated (i.e., either machine-washed or machine-dried using the hot cycle or dry-cleaned) or removed from body contact for at least 72 hours. Fumigation of living areas is unnecessary.

Follow-Up

Pruritus may persist for several weeks. Some experts recommend re-treatment after 1 week for patients who are still symptomatic; other experts recommend re-treatment only if live mites are observed. Patients who do not respond to the recommended treatment should be retreated with an alternative regimen.

Management of Sex Partners and Household Contacts

Both sexual and close personal or household contacts within the preceding month should be examined and treated.

Management of Outbreaks in Communities, Nursing Homes, and Other Institutional Settings

Scabies epidemics often occur in nursing homes, acute- and chronic-care hospitals, residential facilities, and communities. Control of an epidemic can only be achieved by treatment of the entire population at risk. Epidemics should be managed in consultation with an expert.

Special Considerations

Infants, Young Children, and Pregnant or Lactating Women

Infants, young children, and pregnant or lactating women should not be treated with lindane. They may be treated with permethrin.

HIV Infection

Patients who have uncomplicated scabies and also are infected with HIV should receive the same treatment regimen as those who are HIV-negative. HIV-infected patients and others who are immunosuppressed are at increased risk for Norwegian scabies, a disseminated dermatologic infection. Such patients should be managed in consultation with an expert.

SEXUAL ASSAULT AND STDs

Adults and Adolescents

The recommendations in this report are limited to the identification and treatment of sexually transmitted infections and conditions commonly identified in the management of such infections. The documentation of findings and collection of nonmicrobiologic specimens for forensic purposes and the management of potential pregnancy or physical and psychological trauma are not included. Among sexually active adults, the identification of sexually transmitted infections after an assault is usually more important for the psychological and medical management of the patient than for legal purposes, because the infection could have been acquired before the assault.

Trichomoniasis, BV, chlamydia, and gonorrhea are the most frequently diagnosed infections among women who have been sexually assaulted. Because the prevalence of these STDs is substantial among sexually active women, the presence of these infections after an assault does not necessarily signify acquisition during the assault. Chlamydial and gonococcal infections in women are of special concern because of the possibility of ascending infection. In addition, HBV infection, if transmitted to a woman during an assault, can be prevented by post-exposure administration of hepatitis B vaccine.

Evaluation for Sexually Transmitted Infections

Initial Examination

An initial examination should include the following procedures:

- Cultures for *N. gonorrhoeae* and *C. trachomatis* from specimens collected from any sites of penetration or attempted penetration.

- If chlamydial culture is not available, nonculture tests, particularly the nucleic acid amplification tests, are an acceptable substitute. Nucleic acid amplification tests offer advantages of increased sensitivity if confirmation is available. If a nonculture test is used, a positive test result should be verified with a second test based on a different diagnostic principle. EIA and direct fluorescent antibody are not acceptable alternatives, because false-negative test results occur more often with these nonculture tests, and false-positive test results may occur.

- Wet mount and culture of a vaginal swab specimen for *T. vaginalis* infection. If vaginal discharge or malodor is evident, the wet mount also should be examined for evidence of BV and yeast infection.

- Collection of a serum sample for immediate evaluation for HIV, hepatitis B, and syphilis (see Prophylaxis, Risk for Acquiring HIV Infection and Follow-Up Examination 12 Weeks After Assault).

Follow-Up Examinations

Although it is often difficult for persons to comply with follow-up examinations weeks after an assault, such examinations are essential a) to detect new infections acquired during or after the assault; b) to complete hepatitis B immunization, if indicated; and c) to complete counseling and treatment for other STDs. For these reasons, it is recommended that assault victims be reevaluated at follow-up examinations.

Follow-Up Examination After Assault

Examination for STDs should be repeated 2 weeks after the assault. Because infectious agents acquired through assault may not have produced sufficient concentrations of organisms to result in positive test results at the initial examination, a culture (or cultures), a wet mount, and other tests should be repeated at the 2-week follow-up visit unless prophylactic treatment has already been provided.

Serologic tests for syphilis and HIV infection should be repeated 6, 12, and 24 weeks after the assault if initial test results were negative.

Prophylaxis

Many experts recommend routine preventive therapy after a sexual assault. Most patients probably benefit from prophylaxis because the follow-up of patients who have been sexually assaulted can be difficult, and they may be reassured if offered treatment or prophylaxis for possible infection. The following prophylactic regimen is suggested as preventive therapy:

- Postexposure hepatitis B vaccination (without HBIG) should adequately protect against HBV. Hepatitis B vaccine should be administered to victims of sexual assault at the time of the initial examination. Follow-up doses of vaccine should be administered 1–2 and 4–6 months after the first dose.

- An empiric antimicrobial regimen for chlamydia, gonorrhea, trichomonas, and BV should be administered.

Recommended Regimen

Ceftriaxone 125 mg IM in a single dose,
   PLUS
Metronidazole 2 g orally in a single dose,
   PLUS
Azithromycin 1 g orally in a single dose or **Doxycycline** 100 mg orally twice a day for 7 days.

NOTE: For patients requiring alternative treatments, see the sections in this report that specifically address those agents.

The efficacy of these regimens in preventing gonorrhea, BV, or *C. trachomatis* genitourinary infections after sexual assault has not been evaluated. The clinician might consider counseling the patient regarding the possible benefits, as well as the possibility of toxicity, associated with these treatment regimens, because of possible gastrointestinal side effects with this combination.

Other Management Considerations

At the initial examination and, if indicated, at follow-up examinations, patients should be counseled regarding the following:

- Symptoms of STDs and the need for immediate examination if symptoms occur, and

- Abstinence from sexual intercourse until STD prophylactic treatment is completed.

Risk for Acquiring HIV Infection

Although HIV-antibody seroconversion has been reported among persons whose only known risk factor was sexual assault or sexual abuse, the risk for acquiring HIV infection through sexual assault is low. The overall probability of HIV transmission from an HIV-infected person during a single act of intercourse depends on many factors. These factors may include the type of sexual intercourse (i.e., oral, vaginal, or anal); presence of oral, vaginal or anal trauma; site of exposure to ejaculate; viral load in ejaculate; and presence of an STD.

In certain circumstances, the likelihood of HIV transmission also may be affected by postexposure therapy for HIV with antiretroviral agents. Postexposure therapy with zidovudine has been associated with a reduced risk for HIV infection in a study of health-care workers who had percutaneous exposures to HIV-infected blood. On the basis of these results and the biologic plausibility of the effectiveness of antiretroviral agents in preventing infection, postexposure therapy has been recommended for health-care workers who have percutaneous exposures to HIV. However, whether these findings can be extrapolated to other HIV-exposure situations, including sexual assault, is unknown. A recommendation cannot be made, on the basis of available information, regarding the appropriateness of postexposure antiretroviral therapy after sexual exposure to HIV.

Health-care providers who consider offering postexposure therapy should take into account the likelihood of exposure to HIV, the potential benefits and risks of such therapy, and the interval between the exposure and initiation of therapy. Because timely determination of the HIV-infection status of the assailant is not possible in many sexual assaults, the health-care provider should assess the nature of the assault, any available information about HIV-risk behaviors exhibited by persons who are sexual assailants (e.g., high-risk sexual practices and injecting-drug or crack cocaine use), and the local epidemiology of HIV/AIDS. If antiretroviral postexposure prophylaxis is offered, the following information should be discussed with the patient: a) the unknown efficacy and known toxicities of antiretrovirals, b) the critical need for frequent dosing of medications, c) the close follow-up that is necessary, d) the importance of strict compliance with the recommended therapy, and e) the necessity of immediate initiation of treatment for maximal likelihood of effectiveness. If the patient decides to take postexposure therapy, clinical management of the patient should be implemented according to the guidelines for occupational mucous membrane exposure.

Sexual Assault or Abuse of Children

Recommendations in this report are limited to the identification and treatment of STDs. Management of the psychosocial aspects of the sexual assault or abuse of children is important but is not included in these recommendations.

The identification of sexually transmissible agents in children beyond the neonatal period suggests sexual abuse. However, there are exceptions; for example, rectal or genital infection with *C. trachomatis* among young children may be the result of perinatally acquired infection and may persist for as long as 3 years. In addition, genital warts, BV, and genital mycoplasmas have been diagnosed in children who have been abused and in those not abused. There are several modes by which HBV is transmitted to children; the most common of these is household exposure to persons who have chronic HBV infection.

The possibility of sexual abuse should be considered if no obvious risk factor for infection can be identified. When the only evidence of sexual abuse is the isolation of an organism or the detection of antibodies to a sexually transmissible agent, findings should be confirmed and the implications considered carefully. The evaluation for determining whether sexual abuse has occurred among children who have infections that can be sexually transmitted should be conducted in compliance with expert recommendations by practitioners who have experience and training in the evaluation of abused or assaulted children (29).

Evaluation for Sexually Transmitted Infections

Examinations of children for sexual assault or abuse should be conducted so as to minimize pain and trauma to the child. The decision to evaluate the child for STDs must be made on an individual basis. Situations involving a high risk for STDs and a strong indication for testing include the following:

- A suspected offender is known to have an STD or to be at high risk for STDs (e.g., has multiple sex partners or a history of STD).

- The child has symptoms or signs of an STD or of an infection that can be sexually transmitted.

- The prevalence of STDs in the community is high. Other indications recommended by experts include a) evidence of genital or oral penetration or ejaculation or b) STDs in siblings or other children or adults in the household. If a child has symptoms, signs, or evidence of an infection that might be sexually transmitted, the child should be tested for other common STDs. Obtaining the indicated specimens requires skill to avoid psychological and physical trauma to the child. The clinical manifestations of some STDs are different among children in comparison with adults. Examinations and specimen collections should be conducted by practitioners who have experience and training in the evaluation of abused or assaulted children.

A principal purpose of the examination is to obtain evidence of an infection that is likely to have been sexually transmitted. However, because of the legal and psychosocial consequences of a false-positive diagnosis, only tests with high specificities should be used. The additional cost of such tests and the time required to conduct them are justified.

The scheduling of examinations should depend on the history of assault or abuse. If the initial exposure was recent, the infectious agents acquired through the exposure may not have produced sufficient concentrations of organisms to result in positive test results. A follow-up visit approximately 2 weeks after the most recent sexual exposure should include a repeat physical examination and collection of additional specimens. To allow sufficient time for antibodies to develop, another follow-up visit approximately 12 weeks after the most recent sexual exposure may be necessary to collect sera. A single examination may be sufficient if the child was abused for an extended time period or if the last suspected episode of abuse occurred well before the child received the medical evaluation.

The following recommendation for scheduling examinations is a general guide. The exact timing and nature of follow-up contacts should be determined on an individual basis and should be considerate of the child's psychological and social needs. Compliance with follow-up appointments may be improved when law enforcement personnel or child protective services are involved.

Initial and 2-Week Follow-Up Examinations

During the initial examination and 2-week follow-up examination (if indicated), the following should be performed:

- Visual inspection of the genital, perianal, and oral areas for genital warts and ulcerative lesions.

- Cultures for *N. gonorrhoeae* specimens collected from the pharynx and anus in both boys and girls, the vagina in girls, and the urethra in boys. Cervical specimens are not recommended for prepubertal girls. For boys, a meatal specimen of urethral discharge is an adequate substitute for an intraurethral swab specimen when discharge is present. Only standard culture systems for the isolation of *N. gonorrhoeae* should be used. All presumptive isolates of *N. gonorrhoeae* should be confirmed by at least two tests that involve different principles (e.g., biochemical, enzyme substrate, or serologic methods). Isolates should be preserved in case additional or repeated testing is needed.

- Cultures for *C. trachomatis* from specimens collected from the anus in both boys and girls and from the vagina in girls. Limited information suggests that the likelihood of recovering *Chlamydia* from the urethra of prepubertal boys is too low to justify the trauma involved in obtaining an intraurethral specimen. A urethral specimen should be obtained if urethral discharge is present. Pharyngeal specimens for *C. trachomatis* also are not recommended for either sex because the yield is low, perinatally acquired infection may persist beyond infancy, and culture systems in some laboratories do not distinguish between *C. trachomatis* and *C. pneumoniae*.

  Only standard culture systems for the isolation of *C. trachomatis* should be used. The isolation of *C. trachomatis* should be confirmed by microscopic identification of inclusions by staining with fluorescein-conjugated monoclonal antibody specific for *C. trachomatis*. Isolates should be preserved. Nonculture tests for chlamydia are not sufficiently specific for use in circumstances involving possible child abuse or assault. Data are insufficient to adequately assess the utility of nucleic acid amplification tests in the evaluation of children who might have been sexually abused, but expert opinion suggests these tests may be an alternative if confirmation is available but culture systems for *C. trachomatis* are unavailable.

- Culture and wet mount of a vaginal swab specimen for *T. vaginalis* infection. The presence of clue cells in the wet mount or other signs, such as a positive whiff test, suggests BV in girls who have vaginal discharge. The significance of clue cells or other indicators of BV as an indicator of sexual exposure is unclear. The clinical significance of clue cells or other indicators of BV in the absence of vaginal discharge also is unclear.

- Collection of a serum sample to be evaluated immediately, preserved for subsequent analysis, and used as a baseline for comparison with follow-up serologic tests. Sera should be tested immediately for antibodies to sexually transmitted agents. Agents for which suitable tests are available include *T. pal-*

lidum, HIV, and HBsAg. The choice of agents for serologic tests should be made on a case-by-case basis (see Examination 12 Weeks After Assault). HIV antibodies have been reported in children whose only known risk factor was sexual abuse. Serologic testing for HIV infection should be considered for abused children. The decision to test for HIV infection should be made on a case-by-case basis, depending on likelihood of infection among assailant(s). Data are insufficient concerning the efficacy and safety of postexposure prophylaxis among children. Vaccination for HBV should be recommended if the medical history or serologic testing suggests that it has not been received (see Hepatitis B).

Examination 12 Weeks After Assault

An examination approximately 12 weeks after the last suspected sexual exposure is recommended to allow time for antibodies to infectious agents to develop if baseline tests are negative. Serologic tests for *T. pallidum*, HIV, and HBsAg should be considered. The prevalence of these infections differs substantially by community, and serologic testing depends on whether risk factors are known to be present in the abuser or assailant. In addition, results of HBsAg testing must be interpreted carefully, because HBV also can be transmitted nonsexually. The choice of tests must be made on an individual basis.

Presumptive Treatment

The risk for a child's acquiring an STD as a result of sexual abuse has not been determined. The risk is believed to be low in most circumstances, although documentation to support this position is inadequate.

Presumptive treatment for children who have been sexually assaulted or abused is not widely recommended because girls appear to be at lower risk for ascending infection than adolescent or adult women, and regular follow-up usually can be ensured. However, some children—or their parent(s) or guardian(s)—may be concerned about the possibility of infection with an STD, even if the risk is perceived by the health-care provider to be low. Patient or parental/guardian concerns may be an appropriate indication for presumptive treatment in some settings (i.e., after all specimens relevant to the investigation have been collected).

Reporting

Every state, the District of Columbia, Puerto Rico, Guam, the U.S. Virgin Islands, and American Samoa have laws that require the reporting of child abuse. The exact requirements differ by state, but, generally, if there is reasonable cause to suspect child abuse, it must be reported. Health-care providers should contact their state or local child-protection service agency about child abuse reporting requirements in their areas.

References
1. CDC. Hepatitis B virus: a comprehensive strategy for eliminating transmission in the United States through universal childhood vaccination—recommendations of the Immunization Practices Advisory Committee (ACIP). MMWR 1991;40(No. RR-13).
2. CDC. Prevention of hepatitis A through active or passive immunization: recommendations of the Advisory Committee on Immunization Practices (ACIP). MMWR 1996;45(No. RR-15).
3. CDC. Sexually transmitted diseases clinical practice guidelines, 1991. Atlanta: US Department of Health and Human Services, Public Health Service, CDC, 1991.

4. Hatcher RA, Trussell J, Stewart F, et al. Contraceptive technology. 16th ed. New York: Irvington Publishers, 1994.

5. CDC. Technical guidance on HIV counseling. MMWR 1993;42(No. RR-2):11–7.

6. American Academy of Pediatric s/American College of Obstetricians and Gynecologists. Guidelines for perinatal care. 3rd ed. Elk Grove Village, IL: American Academy of Pediatrics/American College of Obstetricians and Gynecologists, 1992.

7. U.S. Preventive Services Task Force. Guide to clinical preventive services. 2nd ed. Baltimore: Williams and Wilkins, 1996.

8. American College of Obstetricians and Gynecologists. Gonorrhea and chlamydial infections. Washington, DC: American College of Obstetricians and Gynecologists, March 1994. (ACOG technical bulletin, no. 190).

9. CDC. Recommendations for the prevention and management of *Chlamydia trachomatis* infections, 1993. MMWR 1993;42(No. RR-12).

10. CDC. 1997 USPHS/IDSA guidelines for the prevention of opportunistic infections in persons infected with human immunodeficiency virus. MMWR 1997;46(No. RR-12).

11. Agency for Health Care Policy and Research. Evaluation and management of early HIV infection. Rockville, MD: US Department of Health and Human Services, Public Health Service, 1994; AHCPR publication no. 94-0572. (Clinical practice guidelines, no. 7).

12. CDC. Testing for antibodies to human immunodeficiency virus type 2 in the United States. MMWR 1992;41(No. RR-12).

13. CDC. Purified protein derivative (PPD)-tuberculin anergy and HIV infection: guidelines for anergy testing and management of anergic persons at risk of tuberculosis. MMWR 1991;40(No. RR-5):27–33.

14. CDC. The use of preventive therapy for tuberculous infection in the United States: recommendations of the Advisory Committee for Elimination of Tuberculosis. MMWR 1990;39(No. RR-8):9–12.

15. CDC. Management of persons exposed to multidrug-resistant tuberculosis. MMWR 1992;41(No. RR-11):59–71.

16. Carpenter CCJ, Fischl MA, Hammer SM, et al. Antiretroviral therapy for HIV infection in 1997: updated recommendations of the International AIDS Society—USA Panel. JAMA 1997;277: 1962–9.

17. CDC. Recommendations for prophylaxis against *Pneumocystis carinii* pneumonia for adults and adolescents infected with human immunodeficiency virus: U.S. Public Health Service Task Force on Antipneumocystis Prophylaxis for Patients with Human Immunodeficiency Virus Infection. MMWR 1992;41(No. RR-4).

18. CDC. 1995 Revised guidelines for prophylaxis against *Pneumocystis carinii* pneumonia for children infected with or perinatally exposed to human immunodeficiency virus. MMWR 1995;44(No. RR-4).

19. Committee on Infectious Diseases, American Academy of Pediatrics. Report of the Committee on Infectious Diseases. 22nd ed. Elk Grove Village, IL: American Academy of Pediatrics, 1991.

20. CDC. Recommendations of the Advisory Committee on Immunization Practices (ACIP): use of vaccines and immune globulins in persons with altered immunocompetence. MMWR 1993;42(No. RR-4).

21. CDC. U.S. Public Health Service recommendations for human imm unodeficiency virus counseling and voluntary testing for pregnant women. MMWR 1995;44(No. RR-7).

22. CDC. Recommendations of the U.S. Public Health Service Task Force on the Use of Zidovudine to Reduce Perinatal Transmission of Human Immunodeficiency Virus. MMWR 1994;43(No. RR-11).

23. Henry RE, Wegmann JA, Hartle JE, Christopher GW. Successful oral acyclovir desensitization. Ann Allergy 1993;70:386–8.

24. Wendel GD Jr, Stark BJ, Jamison RB, Molina RD, Sullivan TJ. Penicillin allergy and desensitization in serious infections during pregnancy. N Engl J Med 1985;312:1229–32.

25. Saxon A, Beall GN, Rohr AS, Adelman DC. Immediate hypersensitivity reactions to beta-lactam antibiotics [Clinical conference]. Ann Intern Med 1987;107:204–15.

26. Pearlman MD, Yashar C, Ernst S, Solomon W. An incremental dosing protocol for women with severe vaginal trichomoniasis and adverse reactions to metronidazole. Am J Obstet Gynecol 1996;174:934–6.

27. National Cancer Institute Workshop. The 1988 Bethesda System for reporting cervical/vaginal cytological diagnoses. JAMA 1989;262:931–4.
28. Kurman RJ, Henson DE, Herbst AL, Noller KL, Schiffman MH, National Cancer Institute Workshop. Interim guidelines for management of abnormal cervical cytology. JAMA 1994;271:1866–9.
29. Committee on Child Abuse and Neglect, American Academy of Pediatrics. Guidelines for the evaluation of sexual abuse of children. Pediatrics 1991;87:254–60.

Neither the CDC nor the U.S. Department of Health and Human Services endorses any particular organization or its activities, products, or services. To order other titles from International Medical Publishing, see your local bookseller or order by mail:

Title	ISBN	Price	Quantity	Subtotal
1998 Guidelines Sexually Transmitted Diseases Centers for Disease Control and Prevention	1-883205-42-5	$7.95	_____	_____
JNC VI High Blood Pressure National Institutes of Health	1-883205-42-5	$8.95	_____	_____
Clinician's Handbook of Preventive Services, 2nd edition U.S. Public Health Service	1-883205-32-8	$20.00	_____	_____
Guide to Clinical Preventive Services, 2nd edition United States Preventive Services Task Force	1-883205-13-1	$24.00	_____	_____
Physical Activity and Health A Report of the Surgeon General	1-883205-31-X	$17.00	_____	_____
Subtotal				_____
Shipping and Handling $4.00 per book		$4.00		_____
Total				_____

Send to:
> International Medical Publishing
> 13017 Wisteria Drive, #313
> Germantown, MD 20874

Name:
Address:

Phone:
e-mail:
Please include check or for Mastercard/VISA, please include expiration date.

Or place orders on the web at *http://www.intlmedpub.com*